Kinn's The Administrative Medical Assistant

Thirteenth Edition

Deborah Proctor, EdD, RN
Adjunct Faculty Member
Butler County Community College
Butler, Pennsylvania

Brigitte Niedzwiecki, RN, MSN, RMA
Medical Assistant Program Director & Instructor
Chippewa Valley Technical College
Eau Claire, Wisconsin

Julie Pepper, BS, CMA (AAMA)
Medical Assistant Instructor
Chippewa Valley Technical College
Eau Claire, Wisconsin

Payel Bhattacharya Madero, MBA, RHIT
Adjunct Faculty
California State University, Fullerton
Fullerton, California

ELSEVIER

ELSEVIER

3251 Riverport Lane
St. Louis, Missouri 63043

Notices

Knowledge and best practice in this field are constantly changing. As new research and experience broaden our understanding, changes in research methods, professional practices, or medical treatment may become necessary.

Practitioners and researchers must always rely on their own experience and knowledge in evaluating and using any information, methods, compounds, or experiments described herein. In using such information or methods they should be mindful of their own safety and the safety of others, including parties for whom they have a professional responsibility.

With respect to any drug or pharmaceutical products identified, readers are advised to check the most current information provided (i) on procedures featured or (ii) by the manufacturer of each product to be administered, to verify the recommended dose or formula, the method and duration of administration, and contraindications. It is the responsibility of practitioners, relying on their own experience and knowledge of their patients, to make diagnoses, to determine dosages and the best treatment for each individual patient, and to take all appropriate safety precautions.

To the fullest extent of the law, neither the Publisher nor the authors, contributors, or editors assume any liability for any injury and/or damage to persons or property as a matter of products liability, negligence or otherwise, or from any use or operation of any methods, products, instructions, or ideas contained in the material herein.

Content Strategist: Jennifer Janson
Content Development Specialist: Rebecca Leenhouts
Publishing Services Manager: Hemamalini Rajendrababu
Project Manager: Manchu Mohan
Cover Designer: Muthukumaran Thangaraj

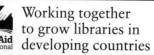

Printed in the United States of America

Last digit is the print number: 9 8 7 6 5 4 3 2 1

To the Student

This study guide was created to help you to achieve the objectives of each chapter in *your text* and to establish a solid base of knowledge in medical assisting. Completing the exercises in each chapter in this guide will help reinforce the material studied in the textbook and learned in class.

STUDY HINTS FOR ALL STUDENTS

Ask Questions!

There are no stupid questions. If you do not know something or are not sure about it, you need to find out. Other people may be wondering the same thing, but are too shy to ask. The answer could be a matter of life or death for your patient. That is certainly more important than feeling embarrassed about asking a question.

CHAPTER OBJECTIVES

At the beginning of each chapter in the textbook are learning objectives that you should have mastered by the time you have finished studying that chapter. Write these objectives in your notebook, leaving a blank space after each. Fill in the answers as you find them while reading the chapter. Review to make sure your answers are correct and complete. Use these answers when you study for tests. You should also do this for separate course objectives that your instructor has listed in your class syllabus.

Vocabulary

At the beginning of each chapter in the textbook are vocabulary terms that you will encounter as you read the chapter. These terms are in bold type the first time they appear in the chapter.

Summary of Learning Objectives

Use the Summary of Learning Objectives at the end of each chapter in the textbook to help you review for exams.

Reading Hints

As you read each chapter in the textbook, look at the subject headings to learn what each section is about. Read first for the general meaning and then reread parts you did not understand. It may help to read those parts aloud. Carefully read the information given in each table and study each figure and its legend.

Concepts

While studying, put difficult concepts into your own words to determine whether you understand them. Check this understanding with another student or the instructor. Write these concepts in your notebook.

Class Notes

When taking lecture notes in class, leave a large margin on the left side of each notebook page and write only on right-hand pages, leaving all left-hand pages blank. Look over your lecture notes soon after each class while your memory is fresh. Fill in missing words, complete sentences and ideas, and underline key phrases, definitions, and concepts. At the top of each page, write the topic of that page. In the left margin, write the key word for that part of your notes. On the opposite left-hand page, write a summary or outline that combines material from the textbook and the lecture. These can be your study notes for review.

Study Groups

Form a study group with other students so that you can help one another. Practice speaking and reading aloud. Ask questions about material you find unclear. Work together to find answers.

ADDITIONAL STUDY HINTS FOR ENGLISH AS A SECOND LANGUAGE (ESL) STUDENTS

Vocabulary

If you find a nontechnical word you do not know (e.g., drowsy), try to guess its meaning from the sentence (e.g., with electrolyte imbalance, the patient may feel fatigued and drowsy). If you are not sure of the meaning or if it seems particularly important, look it up in the dictionary.

Vocabulary Notebook

Keep a small alphabetized notebook or address book in your pocket or purse. Write down new nontechnical words you read or hear along with their meanings and pronunciations. Write each word under its initial letter so that you can find it easily, as in a dictionary. For words you do not know or for words that have a different meaning in medical assisting, write down how each word is used and how it is pronounced. Look up the meanings of these words in a dictionary or ask your instructor or first-language buddy (see the following section). Then write the different meanings or uses that you have found in your book, including the medical assisting meaning. Continue to add new words as you discover them.

First-Language Buddy

English as a second language (ESL) students should find a first-language buddy—another student who is a native speaker of English and who is willing to answer questions about word meanings, pronunciations, and culture. Maybe, in turn, your buddy would like to learn about your language and culture; this could be useful for his or her medical assisting career.

Contents

1 Competency Based Education and the Medical Assistant Student

VOCABULARY REVIEW

Match the following terms and definitions.

1. _____ The constant practice of considering all aspects of a situation when deciding what to believe or what to do

2. _____ The way an individual looks at information and sees it as real

3. _____ The manner in which an individual perceives and processes information to learn new material

4. _____ The way an individual internalizes new information and makes it his or her own

5. _____ The process of thinking about new information so you can create new ways of learning

6. _____ Sensitivity to the individual needs and reactions of patients

7. _____ Mastery of the knowledge, skills, and behaviors that are expected of the entry-level medical assistant

8. _____ A learning device, such as an image, rhyme, or figure of speech, that is used to assist in remembering information

a. Learning style

b. Reflection

c. Processing

d. Empathy

e. Competencies

f. Perceiving

g. Critical thinking

h. Mnemonic

SKILLS AND CONCEPTS

1. Explain the concept of competency-based education. What are the advantages of this method of learning for students who have to learn a large number of skills?

_____

_____

_____

_____

2. What are the core entry-level competencies required by programs that have or are seeking Commission on Accreditation of Allied Health Education Programs (CAAHEP) accreditation?

a. _____

b. _____

c. _____

d. _____

e. _____

f. _____

g. _____

h. _____

1

i. _____

j. _____

3. The Accrediting Bureau of Health Education Schools (ABHES) also focuses curriculum requirements on student competency achievement with the following eleven areas of study:

a. _____

b. _____

c. _____

d. _____

e. _____

f. _____

g. _____

h. _____

i. _____

j. _____

k. _____

4. What do these national standards mean to the medical assistant student?

_____

_____

_____

5. Describe the advantages of a competency-based education for adult learners.

_____

_____

_____

6. What are portfolios and how can they be used in competency-based programs?

_____

_____

_____

7. Discuss the four myths about stress.

a. _____

b. _____

c. _____

d. _____

8. What is the difference between adaptive and nonadaptive coping mechanisms?

_____

_____

_____

9. List and discuss three examples of both adaptive and nonadaptive coping mechanisms.

_____

_____

_____

_____

_____

_____

10. List five time-management skills.

a. _____

b. _____

c. _____

d. _____

e. _____

11. Which of these skills do you think will require the most effort on your road to becoming a medical assistant? How can you better prepare yourself for the challenges ahead?

_____

_____

_____

12. Describe five strategies for breaking the cycle of procrastination.

a. _____

b. _____

c. _____

d. _____

e. _____

13. What barriers cause you to procrastinate? How can you prepare yourself to avoid procrastination?

_____

_____

_____

True or False: Indicate which statements are true (T) and which are false (F).

14. _____ The best way to deal with conflict situations is through open, honest, assertive communication.

15. _____ The first step in conflict management is examination of the pros and cons.

16. _____ Conflicts should be resolved immediately.

17. _____ Sometimes you will not be able to solve problems, or a conflict may not be important enough for you to act to change the situation.

18. _____ It is best if you attempt to solve the conflict in a private place at a prescheduled time.

Chapter **1** **Competency Based Education and the Medical Assistant Student**

19. _____ You need to understand the problem and gather as much information about the situation as possible before you decide to act.

20. _____ As a future member of the healthcare team, you will frequently face problems and conflict.

21. _____ We are born either assertive or passive, and there is nothing we can do to change those behaviors.

22. _____ Assertive communication will get you what you want.

23. _____ A person who responds to conflict passively is truly not bothered by the situation.

24. _____ Nonassertive individuals ultimately may respond with anger or an emotional outburst if pushed too far.

25. _____ Aggressive individuals ignore the needs of others.

Briefly answer the following questions.

26. Describe four different nonassertive behaviors.

    a. _____

    b. _____

    c. _____

    d. _____

27. Describe four different aggressive behaviors that should not be used in professional communication.

    a. _____

    b. _____

    c. _____

    d. _____

28. Explain the process of developing and delivering an assertive message that can be used in professional communication.

    _____

    _____

    _____

29. Examine your own note-taking ability. Review the note-taking strategies described in Chapter 1 and record the ideas you plan to incorporate into your academic goals for this term.

    _____

    _____

    _____

30. Describe how you could use mind maps to help you learn complicated material.

    _____

    _____

    _____

31. Choose three study skills from your reading and describe how you think they will help you learn.

a. _____

b. _____

c. _____

32. What test-taking strategies might help you improve your scores?

_____

_____

_____

33. Describe what it means to be a critical thinker.

_____

_____

_____

34. Identify four items that you could include in a comprehensive portfolio.

a. _____

b. _____

c. _____

d. _____

35. How can tables and graphs be helpful in analyzing healthcare results?

_____

_____

_____

36. Summarize how to analyze a graph.

_____

_____

_____

CASE STUDIES

Read the case studies and answer the questions.

1. Dr. Weaver is running late seeing patients this afternoon. Sara Kline has been waiting in the examination room for Dr. Weaver for 30 minutes. She peeks her head out of the examination room doorway and demands to know what is taking so long. How should you, the medical assistant, approach this patient? How do you calm her down and explain the physician's situation without compromising other patients' confidentiality? What are some things you can do for the patient to make the wait not seem so long?

_____

_____

_____

2. Victoria Graham, a 68-year-old woman with diabetic retinopathy, arrives today for diabetes disease management education. How might the medical assistant approach Ms. Graham's learning style? What are some possible barriers, and how can the medical assistant help Ms. Graham overcome them?

_____

_____

_____

3. You have been working with another student to prepare for your next examination. The student asks to borrow your notes but has yet to return them so you can study for the examination. You are usually a nonassertive person, but you know that you have to get your notes back or you will not do well on the test. How can you formulate an assertive message? Summarize the steps to take and exactly what "I" message you will deliver.

_____

_____

_____

WORKPLACE APPLICATIONS

1. You are the office manager for a busy primary care practice. Over the past week, you have noticed that one of your employees has been at least 15 minutes late every day. Should you approach this employee? If so, how would you manage the situation? What are the main points you would want to stress to this employee? Are there any consequences? What follow-up, if any, should be done?

2. Healthcare practices are extremely busy and must deal with many daily demands. How should one prepare for proper time management? Why is it necessary to prioritize tasks? What are some ideas the medical assistant can use to get the most out of the day and stay organized?

3. Connie is the manager of a busy family practice. The insurance clerk has complained that the receptionist takes too many smoking breaks and accepts too many personal calls while at work. What type of information should Connie obtain before approaching the receptionist? How should this situation be handled? Where? Who should be present?

4. After being on vacation for a week, Laura returns to work to find her desk piled high with a number of tasks. Laura decides to get organized and make a list of the items that need attention. Prioritize the following tasks from "most important and urgent" to "needs to be done later today" and "may be done later this week." Explain your answers.

   a. Make a staff schedule for next week.

   b. Pull patients' charts for the laboratory results the office received this morning for the physician's review.

   c. Call and order immunization vaccines (the staff has informed you they are on the last vial).

   d. Call and confirm the patient appointments for tomorrow.

   e. Order general stock supplies (e.g., bandages, gauze, needles, and sharps containers).

   f. Review the insurance reimbursements the practice received for last month and address any claims that have not been paid.

   g. File charts.

   h. Edit the physician's schedule for a meeting scheduled next month.

INTERNET ACTIVITY

Refer to the learning styles inventory developed by Barbara A. Soloman and Richard M. Felder from North Carolina State University at www.engr.ncsu.edu/learningstyles/ilsweb.html. Complete the Index of Learning Styles Questionnaire. What did you think about the process? Did you learn anything about yourself and how you prefer to learn? Discuss the Index with your class.

2 The Medical Assistant and the Healthcare Team

VOCABULARY REVIEW

Fill in the blanks with the correct vocabulary terms from this chapter.

1. A nurse sees several patients in a hospital emergency department and determines which patient is the most ill and should be seen by the physician first. The process the nurse is using is called _____.

2. A new hospital contacts The Joint Commission (formerly JCAHO) to begin the _____ process, which verifies that the facility meets or exceeds standards.

3. Dr. Margolis practices _____ medicine, which treats disease through the use of remedies such as medications and surgery. Most of the physicians in the United States practice this type of medicine.

4. Chiropractic care is one of the most common fields of _____, which uses a variety of treatment methods that are not generally considered part of conventional medicine.

5. _____ is the process by which something becomes harmful or unusable by contact with something unclean.

6. Osteopathic physicians are trained to consider all factors about the patient when deciding on treatment plans. This approach is called _____ care.

7. _____ care provides medical, psychological, and spiritual support to terminally ill patients and their families.

8. The Joint Commission uses standard _____ to determine whether patients are receiving quality care in an institution that is seeking initial or continued accreditation.

9. A medical assistant who does not meet the expected standard of care may be charged with professional _____.

10. Chiropractors treat slight misalignments of the spine, which are called _____.

SKILLS AND CONCEPTS

1. Complete the following table that outlines medical pioneers and their achievements.

Name	Achievement
	Father of modern anatomy—Wrote first anatomy book
	Discovered the circulatory system
Anton van Leeuwenhoek	
	Founder of scientific surgery
Edward Jenner	
	Developed smallpox vaccine

7

Name	Achievement
	First physician to recommend hand washing to prevent puerperal fever; believed there was a connection between performing autopsies and then delivering babies
Florence Nightingale	
	Established the American Red Cross
Elizabeth Blackwell	
	Father of bacteriology and preventive medicine—developed pasteurization and the connection between germs and disease
Joseph Lister	
Robert Koch	
	Proved that yellow fever was transmitted by mosquito bites while serving in the U.S. Army in Cuba
	Injected chemicals for the first time to treat disease (syphilis)
	Discovered the x-ray
Marie Curie	
Alexander Fleming	
	Developed the oral live-virus vaccine for polio 10 years after Salk developed the first injected vaccine
Virginia Apgar	
Jonas Salk	
	Performed the first human heart transplant
	Pioneered the technique of in-vitro fertilization (IVF)
	AIDS research pioneer

2. Choose one of these medical pioneers and do further research on his or her contribution to medicine. How does this individual's work affect medicine today?

_____

_____

_____

Spell out the following acronyms and explain their primary responsibility for the health of citizens of the United States.

3. OSHA

_____

4. HHS

_____

5. CDC

_____

6. NIH

_____

7. Describe how the profession of medical assisting began. Why are medical assistants defined as multiskilled health-care workers?

_____

_____

_____

8. Summarize the history of the American Association of Medical Assistants (AAMA) and explain what impact this medical assisting professional organization has on the training and certification of medical assistants today.

_____

_____

_____

9. What are some of the differences between the AAMA and American Medical Technologists (AMT)?

_____

_____

_____

10. Is the National Healthcareer Association (NHA) involved in medical assistant program curriculum development or accreditation? What service does this company provide?

_____

_____

_____

11. List five clinical and five administrative skills that are part of the job description for an entry-level medical assistant.

    Clinical skills include:

    a. _____

    b. _____

    c. _____

    d. _____

    e. _____

    Administrative skills include:

    f. _____

    g. _____

    h. _____

    i. _____

    j. _____

Use the appropriate terms to complete these sentences.

12. A(n) _____ is trained to locate subluxations of the spine and repair them using x-ray examinations and adjustments.

13. _____ physicians, or DOs, complete requirements similar to those for MDs to graduate and practice medicine.

14. The professional who is trained and licensed to examine the eyes, test visual acuity, and treat defects of vision by prescribing correctional lenses is called a(n) _____.

15. A(n) _____ is educated in the care of the feet, including surgical treatment.

16. _____ and medical laboratory technicians perform diagnostic testing on blood, body fluids, and other types of specimens to assist the physician in obtaining a diagnosis.

17. _____ provide direct patient care services under the supervision of licensed physicians and are trained to diagnose and treat patients as directed by the physician.

18. _____ are registered nurses who provide anesthetics to patients during procedures performed by surgeons, physicians, dentists, or other qualified healthcare professionals.

19. _____ assist patients in regaining their mobility and improving their strength and range of motion, which may have been impaired by an accident or injury or as a result of disease.

20. Explain the role of the hospitalist.

_____

_____

_____

21. Hospitals are classified according to the type of care and services they provide to patients. Describe the three different levels of hospitalized care:

   a. _____

   b. _____

   c. _____

22. Define a patient-centered medical home (PCMH) and its five core functions and attributes.

   a. _____

   b. _____

   c. _____

   d. _____

   e. _____

23. What is the difference between scope of practice and standards of care?

_____

_____

_____

24. Identify five practices that are beyond the scope of practice of medical assistants.

a. _____

b. _____

c. _____

d. _____

e. _____

Allied Healthcare Occupations and Licensed Medical Professions

Match the following descriptions with the appropriate healthcare occupation.

1. _____ Provides services such as injury prevention, assessment, and rehabilitation

2. _____ Is qualified to implement exercise programs designed to reverse or minimize debilitation and enhance the functional capacity of medically stable patients

3. _____ Practices medicine under the direction and responsible supervision of a medical doctor or doctor of osteopathy

4. _____ Performs diagnostic examinations and therapeutic interventions of the heart or blood vessels, both invasive and noninvasive

5. _____ Assists licensed pharmacists by performing duties that do not require the expertise of a pharmacist

6. _____ Assists in developing and implementing the anesthesia care plan

7. _____ Helps to improve patient mobility, relieve pain, and prevent or limit permanent physical disabilities

8. _____ Helps patients use their leisure in ways that enhance health, functional abilities, independence, and quality of life

9. _____ Identifies patients who have hearing, balance, and related ear problems

10. _____ Integrates and applies the principles from the science of food, nutrition, biochemistry, food management, and behavior to achieve and maintain health

11. _____ Evaluates, treats, and manages patients of all ages with respiratory illnesses and other cardiopulmonary disorders

12. _____ Evaluates disorders of vision, eye movement, and eye alignment

13. _____ Performs routine and standardized tests in blood center and transfusion services

14. _____ Uses equipment that produces sound waves, resulting in images of internal structures

15. _____ Uses the nuclear properties of radioactive and stable nuclides to make diagnostic evaluations of the anatomic or physiologic conditions of the body

a. Audiologist

b. Diagnostic cardiovascular technologist

c. Therapeutic recreation specialist

d. Physical therapist

e. Pharmacy technician

f. Dietetic technician

g. Anesthesiology assistant

h. Blood bank technology specialist

i. Diagnostic medical sonographer

j. Kinesiotherapist

k. Occupational therapist

l. Orthoptist

m. Physician assistant

n. Surgical technologist

o. Respiratory therapist

p. Athletic trainer

q. Medical technologist

r. Emergency medical technician

s. Nuclear medicine technologist

16. _____ Helps prepare patients for surgery and maintain the sterile field in the surgical suite, making sure all members of the surgical team follow sterile technique

17. _____ Assists in helping patients compensate for loss of function

18. _____ Performs diagnostic testing on blood, body fluids, and other types of specimens to assist the provider in arriving at a diagnosis

19. _____ Provides medical care to patients who have suffered an injury or illness outside the hospital setting

CASE STUDIES

Match the following patients with the physician who should treat them. The specialties are based on the divisions of medicine recognized by the American Board of Medical Specialties. Write the corresponding letter for the physician on the blank next to the patient's name.

1. _____ Mr. West has complained of problems with excessive gas and bloating after meals. He also has some pain in his lower abdominal area.

2. _____ Ms. Jindra has suffered from severe acne most of her adult life. She hopes to find a treatment that will give her more confidence in her appearance.

3. _____ The results of Ms. Robles's amniocentesis are abnormal, and her obstetrician suspects that she may be carrying a child who will be born with a birth defect.

4. _____ Ms. O'Neal is pregnant with her first child.

5. _____ Ms. Sklaar had gastric bypass surgery 2 years ago and now wants to undergo abdominoplasty to remove excess skin.

6. _____ Mr. Taylor experiences pain in his left eye when he is exposed to bright sunlight. He is concerned because his mother and grandmother both lost their eyesight in their later years.

7. _____ Jack Monroe is the lead singer for a popular rock band. He experienced laryngitis during a world tour and needs to see a physician quickly to help him get back on the road.

8. _____ Sarah is 1 year old and needs several immunizations.

9. _____ Jimmie suffers from asthma related to reactions that occur when he is around grass, shrubs, and some animals.

10. _____ Mrs. Downey had a stroke and needs surgery to remove a small clot that has lodged in her brain.

11. _____ Andrea is having a hysterectomy and will be given a general anesthetic. While in the hospital, she meets the physician who will administer the anesthetic during surgery.

12. _____ Mrs. Ballard had an ovarian cyst, which was removed after a visit to the emergency department. She received a bill later from the physician who evaluated the cyst for malignancies.

a. Dr. Stayer, pediatrician

b. Dr. Quincy, pathologist

c. Dr. Haskins, geneticist

d. Dr. Marrs, urologist

e. Dr. Cantrell, neurologist

f. Dr. DuBois, ophthalmologist

g. Dr. Gleaton, anesthesiologist

h. Dr. Kirkham, otolaryngologist

i. Dr. Jones, general surgeon

j. Dr. Faught, internal medicine

k. Dr. Martin, primary care physician

l. Dr. Rowinski, neurosurgeon

m. Dr. Antonetti, plastic surgeon

n. Dr. Jackson, colorectal surgeon

o. Dr. Tips, allergist/immunologist

p. Dr. Roberts, radiologist

q. Dr. Skylar, dermatology

r. Dr. Burns, emergency medicine

s. Dr. True, obstetrics/gynecology

t. Dr. Williams, thoracic surgeon

Chapter **2** **The Medical Assistant and the Healthcare Team**

13. _____ Ms. Harris had several polyps in her gastrointestinal tract. She was referred for surgery by her primary care physician.

14. _____ Ms. Richardson has had migraine headaches for about 6 months. Her primary care physician thinks she should see this specialist.

15. _____ Bobbie broke his arm and was taken to the emergency department. X-ray films were taken, and a physician read them.

16. _____ Mr. Oldman periodically suffers from kidney stones and may need surgery.

17. _____ Rhonda was taken to the emergency department after a car accident.

18. _____ Mr. Anton contacted a physician for removal of a minor cyst on his back.

19. _____ The entire Blair family sees one physician.

20. _____ Mr. Saxton will have surgery tonight to treat a punctured lung.

1. Rebecca is a new employee at the Blackburn Clinic. She recently graduated from an accredited medical assistant school and completed her externship in a primary care facility. She enjoys the variety of patients who come to the office and respects the providers for their dedication to the art and science of medicine. The physicians with whom Rebecca works are strong proponents of continuing education, and they want Rebecca to attend no fewer than two seminars each year.

   Research the history of primary care and answer these questions.

   a. What types of patients are seen in a primary care practice?

   _____

   _____

   _____

   b. What educational background is required to become a primary care physician?

   _____

   _____

   _____

   c. What are some of the common illnesses that present in a primary care facility?

   _____

   _____

   _____

   d. What age groups are cared for by primary care physicians? Why are primary care physicians considered "gatekeepers"?

   _____

   _____

   _____

2. What does it mean to operate as a patient navigator in the facility where you are employed? Why are medical assistants who are skilled in both administrative and clinical skills ideally suited to help patients navigate complex healthcare systems? How could you help the patient described below?

Mrs. Kate Glasgow is an 82-year-old patient in the family practice where you work. Mrs. Glasgow recently suffered a mild cerebrovascular accident (CVA) and her son is trying to help coordinate her care. Mrs. Glasgow does not understand when or how to take her new medications, she is concerned about whether her health insurance will cover the cost of frequent clinic appointments and assistive devices, she doesn't understand how to prepare for magnetic resonance imaging (MRI) the doctor ordered, and she dislikes having to comply with getting blood drawn every week.

_____

_____

_____

WORKPLACE APPLICATION OPTIONS

Complete one or more of these activities and share your results with the class if appropriate.

1. You are employed by a primary care physician who is investigating the possibility of forming a patient-centered medical home with other practitioners and allied health professionals in the community. Refer to the Department of Health and Human Services PCMH Resource Center at http://pcmh.ahrq.gov/. Research the meaning of a PCMH and review the research that supports the PCMH model of care. What did you learn? Share this information with your class.

2. Investigate the hospital systems in your community or region. Choose one system and share its components with the class, explaining the services that each entity offers.

INTERNET ACTIVITY OPTIONS

Choose one or more of these activities and share your results with the class if appropriate.

1. Choose one of the early medical pioneers discussed in this chapter and research him or her using the Internet. After conducting the research, write a report and present the person to the class. Be creative with the presentation by using PowerPoint or some type of audiovisual equipment.

2. Research the two primary professional medical assisting organizations, the AAMA and the AMT. What are their differences? What services does each offer professional medical assistants?

3. Research scope of practice laws in your state that pertain to medical assistants. Does your state have a scope of practice law? If not, what does that mean for the parameters of your work?

3 Professional Behavior in the Workplace

VOCABULARY REVIEW

Fill in the blanks with the correct vocabulary terms from this chapter.

1. Roberta _____ the notes from the last staff meeting to all employees.

2. A few of the _____ that the professional medical assistant should possess include loyalty, initiative, and courtesy.

3. Kristen has a pleasant _____ when working with patients.

SKILLS AND CONCEPTS

1. List and describe six attributes of the professional medical assistant.

   a. _____

   b. _____

   c. _____

   d. _____

   e. _____

   f. _____

2. What methods can the medical assistant use to treat others with courtesy and respect?

   _____

   _____

   _____

   _____

3. Dependability and honesty are critical components to earning the trust and respect of others. How can an entry-level medical assistant perform his or her duties with responsibility, integrity, and honesty?

   _____

   _____

   _____

   _____

4. Summarize three obstructions to professionalism.

   a. _____

   b. _____

   c. _____

17

5. Which of the obstructions to professionalism will be most difficult for you to overcome? Explain why.

_____

_____

_____

_____

6. Describe the important factors that should be considered when you visualize the image of a professional medical assistant.

_____

_____

_____

_____

7. Why is it important for a professional medical assistant to respond to constructive criticism?

_____

_____

_____

_____

8. Which professional attribute is your greatest strength? Which one will require more effort to achieve? Explain why.

_____

_____

_____

_____

9. Define the principles of self-boundaries. How do they relate to the field of medical assisting?

_____

_____

_____

_____

10. Describe four time-management techniques medical assistants can use in the healthcare environment to meet the demands of a busy practice.

    a. _____

    b. _____

    c. _____

    d. _____

11. Define teamwork in your own words.

_____

_____

_____

_____

Name _____ Date _____ Score _____

PROCEDURE 2-1. LOCATE A STATE'S LEGAL SCOPE OF PRACTICE FOR MEDICAL ASSISTANTS

CAAHEP COMPETENCIES: X.P.1.
ABHES COMPETENCIES: 4.f.

TASK: Determine the legal scope of practice for medical assistants employed in your home state.

There is no single definition of the scope of practice for medical assistants throughout the United States, but some states have enacted scope of practice laws covering medical assistant practice. These states include Alaska, Arizona, California, Florida, Georgia, Illinois, Maine, Maryland, Montana, Nevada, New Hampshire, New Jersey, New York, Ohio, South Dakota, Virginia, Washington, and West Virginia. Medical assistants working in those states must refer to the identified roles specified in the law. For those employed in states without scope of practice laws, medical assistant practice is guided by the norms of that particular location, facility policies and procedures, and individual physician employers. In some states, medical assistants are overseen by the board of nursing, whereas in others the board of medicine oversees medical assistants. Make sure you are aware of your state's rules governing medical assistant scope of practice.

Research the scope of practice laws in your state and summarize what you have learned.

EQUIPMENT AND SUPPLIES:
• Computer with Internet access

Standards: Complete the procedure and all critical steps in _____ minutes with a minimum score of 85% within three attempts.

Scoring: Divide the points earned by the total possible points. Failure to perform a critical step indicated by an asterisk (*) results in an unsatisfactory overall score.

Time began _____ Time ended _____ Total minutes: _____

Steps	Possible Points	Attempt 1	Attempt 2	Attempt 3
*1. Google "medical assistant state scope of practice laws" or refer to the American Association of Medical Assistants site at www.aama-ntl.org/employers/state-scope-of-practice-laws.	40	_____	_____	_____
*2. Summarize the scope of medical assistant practice in your state, and give details on where you found this information.	30	_____	_____	_____
*3. Discuss the scope of practice for medical assistants in your home state with your peers.	30	_____	_____	_____

Comments:

Points earned _____ ÷ 100 possible points = Score _____ % Score

Instructor's signature _____

12. What are the benefits of becoming a member of the AAMA?

_____

_____

_____

_____

CASE STUDIES

1. Karen has developed a friendship with her co-worker Angela, who has a wonderful personality but does not always do her fair share of work in the family practice clinic. How can Karen implement the theory of self-boundaries to help her deal with the situation?

_____

_____

_____

_____

2. Martin Smith is a patient who always disrupts the clinic. He constantly complains about everything from the moment he enters until the moment he leaves. Karen is at the desk when he arrives to check out and pay his bill. When she tells him that he has a previous balance from a claim that his insurance did not pay, he argues that Karen filed the claim incorrectly. Karen is not in charge of filing insurance claims and did not handle any part of the claim in question. How can she be courteous to this patient?

_____

_____

_____

_____

3. Karen works in the facility's medical laboratory. She is often asked questions about insurance and billing that she must refer to other personnel. How should Karen efficiently request information or assistance for the patient from other office personnel?

_____

_____

_____

_____

4. Karen and her fiancé ended their relationship last week. How can she deal with personal stressors while she is in the workplace?

_____

_____

_____

_____

5. A patient needs to be scheduled for an outpatient endoscopic examination. When Karen gives the instruction sheet to the patient, she suspects from his reaction that the patient is unable to read. How can Karen professionally handle this situation without causing embarrassment to the patient?

_____

_____

_____

_____

6. You are trying to help a patient, Mr. Chad Fisher, who is very unhappy about having to be scheduled for an MRI because of his chronic back pain. Using professional behaviors, how can you help Mr. Fisher understand the importance of following through with the ordered diagnostic study?

_____

_____

_____

_____

7. You have been asked to complete an insurance form that you have never seen before. You are not sure how to complete two sections of the form. As a professional medical assistant, how should you honestly handle this situation?

_____

_____

_____

_____

WORKPLACE APPLICATIONS

1. *Professionalism* is a word that's often used with regard to medical personnel. What does professionalism mean? Write a report on the meaning of professionalism, highlighting a person you believe is the epitome of professionalism in the medical field. This person could be an instructor, a physician, or some other healthcare worker whom you have come to know. Be specific about the ways professionalism is apparent in this individual's actions and speech.

2. Create a document for an office policy manual that defines and explains how the medical assistant working in the healthcare facility should display professionalism toward patients, co-workers, physicians, and visitors.

INTERNET ACTIVITIES

Complete one or more of these activities and share your results with the class, if appropriate.

1. Find four articles on medical professionalism. What seem to be the primary challenges in attempting to maintain professionalism in medical facilities?

2. Research professionalism requirements for other health professions. Talk about the ways that those requirements are similar to or different from those of a medical assistant. Compare professionalism in the healthcare industry to that in other professions, such as law enforcement or education. Talk about why medical professionalism is so critical.

3. Research the AAMA and AMT online. How can an entry-level medical assistant benefit from becoming a member of these organizations?

Student Name _____ Date_____

AFFECTIVE COMPETENCY: V.A2. DEMONSTRATE THE PRINCIPLES OF SELF-BOUNDARIES

Explanation: Student must achieve a minimum score of 3 in each category to achieve competency.

Personal or self-boundaries are extremely individual. We all determine our physical, emotional, and mental limits and use them to protect ourselves in both our personal and professional lives. Personal boundaries are developed to protect ourselves from being manipulated or used by others. Each individual's personal boundaries help identify them as a particular individual with certain thoughts and feelings that separate them from others. Self-boundaries help identify our uniqueness as individuals.

We must recognize our individual self-boundaries and appreciate their presence in others in order to develop healthy relationships in both our personal and professional lives. In other words, we expect those we live and work with to recognize and understand our personal limits, and at the same time we must respect the self-boundaries displayed by others. Personal boundaries allow us to preserve our integrity and take responsibility for who we are and how we treat others. Even though we have the right to determine our own self-boundaries, we do not have the right to expect that everyone we interact with feels the same way we do.

Awareness of personal boundaries helps us determine the actions and behaviors that we find unacceptable. Healthy self-boundaries make it possible for us to respect our strengths, abilities, and individuality, as well as those of others.

Using the information discussed in the Professional Behavior in the Workplace chapter, role-play with your partner how you would respond if a patient requests your personal telephone number just in case he has questions after office hours.

Scoring Criteria (1 Thru 4)	Excellent Evidence of Learning 4	Adequate Evidence of Learning 3	Limited Evidence of Learning 2	Unacceptable Evidence of Learning 1	Score Attempt 1	Score Attempt 2	Score Attempt 3
Demonstrates the principles of self-boundaries	Student demonstrates the highest level of awareness of self-boundaries	Student demonstrates mastery level of awareness of self-boundaries but does not apply the principles comprehensively	Student is developing competency in awareness of self-boundaries	Student demonstrates the main concepts of awareness of self-boundaries but does not perform them adequately			
Analyzes the situation and synthesizes a resolution	Considers the concept of self-boundaries before reaching a solution	Identifies most of the factors of self-boundaries	Limited recognition of self-boundaries	Fails to identify significant self-boundary factors			
Evaluates the outcome of his or her actions	Assesses the personal and professional response to the situation	Briefly considers the personal and professional response to the situation	Limited consideration of the personal and professional response to the situation	Fails to evaluate the personal and professional response to the situation			

Instructor Comments

4 Therapeutic Communications

VOCABULARY REVIEW

Fill in the blanks with the correct vocabulary terms from this chapter.

1. A comment that large individuals are lazy is an example of a(n) _____.

2. Tiffany is constantly aware of whether there is _____ between her verbal message and her body language.

SKILLS AND CONCEPTS

Part I: Short Answers
Answer the following questions.

1. What are some of the factors that contribute to a patient's first impression of a healthcare facility?

   _____

   _____

   _____

2. Define patient-centered care.

   _____

   _____

   _____

3. How can the medical assistant contribute to positive patient-centered care in a healthcare facility?

   _____

   _____

   _____

4. What are the two types of verbal communication? Explain each and describe what methods can be used to deliver a verbal message.

   _____

   _____

   _____

5. Describe two areas of concern when sending an e-mail or text message.

   _____

   _____

   _____

6. Describe the significance of congruence between a verbal and a nonverbal message. How can you make sure the message you send to a patient or co-worker is congruent?

_____

_____

_____

7. Complete the following table that can be used when observing the nonverbal behaviors of patients.

Area Observed	Observation	Indication
Breathing patterns	Rapid respirations, sighing, shallow thoracic breathing	
Eye patterns	No eye contact, side-to-side movement, looking down at the hands	
Hands	Tapping fingers, cracking knuckles, continuous movement, sweaty palms	
Arm placement	Folded across chest, wrapped around abdomen	
Leg placement	Tension, crossed and/or tucked under, tapping foot, continuous movement	

8. Summarize five positive nonverbal behaviors that the medical assistant can use to enhance the patient's experience in the healthcare setting.

   a. _____

   b. _____

   c. _____

   d. _____

   e. _____

9. Discuss five communication barriers that can result in misunderstanding of the medical assistant's message

   a. _____

   b. _____

   c. _____

   d. _____

   e. _____

10. Explain how the following patient communication barriers might interfere with therapeutic communication in the healthcare setting.

   a. Physical impairment _____

   _____

   b. Language _____

   _____

11. Describe the meaning of stereotyping people and how it can affect therapeutic communication.

   _____

   _____

   _____

12. Explain three factors to consider when communicating with diverse patient groups.

    a. _____

    b. _____

    c. _____

13. Summarize three methods you can use to overcome barriers to communication.

    a. _____

    b. _____

    c. _____

14. Describe the linear communication model that involves the sender of the message, the receiver, and the crucial component of feedback to confirm reception of the message.

    _____

    _____

    _____

15. What is a communication channel? List four examples of possible channels that can be used when sending a message to a receiver.

    _____

    _____

    _____

    _____

16. Active listening techniques are crucial to therapeutic communications. Describe the three components of active listening and give an example of each.

    a. Restatement

    _____

    _____

    b. Reflection

    _____

    _____

    c. Clarification

    _____

    _____

17. Identify three helpful listening guidelines.

    a. _____

    b. _____

    c. _____

18. Summarize how to communicate effectively with children.

    _____

    _____

    _____

19. List three suggestions for effective communication with aging patients.

a. _____

b. _____

c. _____

Part II: Application of Learning

1. How might your personal value system influence your reaction to a diverse population of patients? What do you value most in life? What is important to you? What influences you to act in a certain way? Make a list of three things you value the most. Try to determine why you feel so strongly about those particular things.

_____

_____

_____

_____

_____

2. Label the following questions or statements as either open ended (O) or closed (C).

a. _____ Are you taking blood pressure medication?

b. _____ Are you allergic to aspirin?

c. _____ Would you tell me about your past surgeries?

d. _____ Do you have asthma?

e. _____ What types of attempts have you made to stop smoking?

f. _____ Explain what you feel when your migraines begin.

g. _____ Do you have hospitalization insurance?

h. _____ Do you want a morning or afternoon appointment?

i. _____ How are you feeling today?

j. _____ What type of trouble do you have when swallowing pills?

3. Consider the following scenarios and discuss them with your classmates:

a. While you are gathering a patient's insurance information, the patient tells you that he has tested positive for the human immunodeficiency virus (HIV). Do you think this will affect your therapeutic relationship?

b. An individual with very poor hygiene stops in the office to make an appointment to see the physician. Will this cause a problem with your professional manner?

c. You are told by your office manager that an inmate of the county prison is being brought in this afternoon for an examination. Do you think his status will affect your interaction with the patient?

d. You are attempting to register a 20-year-old patient who brought her two young children with her to the office today. She is a single mother who is pregnant with her third child and receives public assistance. What do you think? Will you have difficulty being empathetic and communicating therapeutically with this young woman?

4. If a non–English-speaking patient comes to the office without an interpreter, what should the medical assistant do?

_____

_____

_____

5. How can the medical assistant put a patient at ease who seems nervous about an office visit or a procedure?

_____

_____

_____

6. Why should the medical assistant avoid the phrase "I know how you feel"?

_____

_____

_____

7. Draw and label Maslow's hierarchy of needs as shown in the text. Explain the importance of each level.

CASE STUDIES

Read the case studies and answer the questions that follow.

1. Simone Lange, 28, was recently diagnosed with an eating disorder and hypotension. She is being seen today to follow up on her recommended diet and medication therapy. Ms. Lange also has issues with her bill and canceled the last two follow-up appointments. She tells the medical assistant who is trying to help her understand her bill that she is just going to quit coming to the doctor because she isn't getting any better and she can't afford it anyway. She is sitting straight up in the chair with her legs crossed and is swinging her leg, periodically chewing her nails, and refuses to make eye contact.
   Communication factors that should be considered in this case include the following:

   a. What nonverbal behaviors are being used by Ms. Lange and how might they be interpreted?

   _____

   _____

   b. Ms. Lange tells the medical assistant she is not following that crazy diet and refuses to make an appointment with the hospital dietitian. What therapeutic communication skills can be used to get more information from Ms. Lange and to reinforce the provider's recommendations?

   _____

   _____

   c. During the discussion Ms. Lange says she stopped taking the medication prescribed by the provider because of the side effects. What communication techniques and therapeutic body language can be used to emphasize the need for Ms. Lange to take her medicine as prescribed?

   _____

   _____

2. Aretha dreads the days that Rahima Bathkar comes to the office. She is a pleasant patient, but Aretha cannot understand her well and feels as if she is not providing Rahima with the care she deserves. She is always worried that she is missing some information the physician needs to know to diagnose and treat the patient properly. Aretha takes extra time with Rahima, but she is concerned because there is no one to interpret for Rahima when she cannot find the right word in her broken English. What can Aretha do to improve communication with Rahima?

   _____

   _____

   _____

Chapter **4** **Therapeutic Communications**

3. Allan and Rebecca Poe are an elderly couple who visit the clinic twice a month for Rebecca's diabetes. Mrs. Poe is blind in one eye and cannot read easily and Mr. Poe has hearing problems. How can the medical assistant improve therapeutic communications with this aging couple?

_____

_____

_____

4. Tommy Lightman approached the office manager because he was concerned about the manner in which Sarah spoke to him in the office. He expressed that Sarah was quite short with him last Tuesday and seemed very distracted as she talked with him in the examination room before the provider came in to treat him. He also said that the provider seemed to spend less time with him that day than usual. Tommy was concerned that he was not wanted in the clinic and wished to have his records sent to another facility. The office manager checks the appointment book and realizes that Tommy was in the office last Tuesday at 11 o'clock, which was the exact time that another patient was being transported to the hospital because of heart failure. How can the office manager manage this difficult situation?

_____

_____

_____

5. Teresa has a difficult time dealing with Orlando Gutierrez. He comes for appointments twice a month and is trying desperately to lose weight. He currently weighs 435 pounds. He is a pleasant person, but Teresa has been raised to believe that those who are overweight are lazy individuals. How might Teresa's personal value system conflict with professionalism in this case? How can she interact with the patient respectfully?

_____

_____

_____

INTERNET ACTIVITIES

1. Investigate therapeutic communications online. Summarize one thing you learned and share it with the class.

_____

_____

_____

2. Search online for sites that outline polite electronic communication methods. What did you learn?

_____

_____

_____

3. Research Maslow's hierarchy of needs. Does this make sense to you? Can you give a personal example of when you were not able to meet the needs of one of the levels? Do you think this knowledge can better help you understand certain patient behaviors? Discuss with the class.

_____

_____

_____

Student Name _____ _____ Date _____

AFFECTIVE COMPETENCIES: V.A1. DEMONSTRATE EMPATHY, ACTIVE LISTENING, AND NONVERBAL COMMUNICATION SKILLS; V.A3. DEMONSTRATE RESPECT FOR INDIVIDUAL DIVERSITY

Explanation: Student must achieve a minimum score of 3 in each category to achieve competency.

Practicing respectful patient care is extremely important when working with a diverse patient population. Empathy is the key to creating a caring, therapeutic environment. Empathy goes beyond sympathy. A medical assistant who is empathetic respects the individuality of the patient and attempts to see the person's health problem through his or her eyes, recognizing the effect of holistic factors on the patient's well-being. Active listening techniques encourage patients to expand on and clarify the content and meaning of their messages. Three processes are involved in active listening: restatement, reflection, and clarification. Much of what we communicate to our patients is conveyed through the use of conscious or unconscious body language. Our nonverbal actions, such as gestures, facial expressions, and mannerisms, express our true feelings. Experts say that more than 90% of communication is nonverbal, in fact. Although the verbal message is an important method of delivering information, the way we deliver those words is how the patient will interpret them.

Many factors influence therapeutic communication with patients and their families, including culture, gender, race, religion, age, economic status, and appearance. For therapeutic communication to be successful, it is essential that the medical assistant be aware of and sensitive to the impact of these factors on patient interactions. Some questions you should consider when communicating with a patient from a diverse background include:

- Is language an issue with your patient?
- Do the patient's culture, ethnic background, or religious beliefs influence the way he or she perceives disease and/or the role of healthcare workers?
- What strategies or techniques might minimize communication problems?
- Are community resources available that could facilitate therapeutic communication?

Approaches for Language Barriers
- Address the patient by his or her last name (e.g., Mrs. Martinez, Mr. Nguyen).
- Be courteous and use a formal approach to communication.
- Use gestures, tone of voice, facial expressions, and eye contact to emphasize appropriate parts of the discussion.
- Integrate pictures, handouts, models, and other aids that visually depict the material.
- Monitor the patient's body language—especially facial expression—for understanding or confusion.
- Use simple, everyday words as much as possible.
- Demonstrate all procedures and have the patient return the demonstration to check for understanding.
- Give the patient written instructions, preferably in their native language, for all procedures and treatments.
- Involve family members in care or use an interpreter.

Using the following case study from the Therapeutic Communications chapter, role-play with your partner how you would apply respect for diversity in this situation that requires extensive therapeutic communication techniques. Demonstrate empathy, active listening, and nonverbal communication skills while performing the role-play exercise.

Mrs. Maria Rodriquez, a 61-year-old Hispanic patient, was recently diagnosed with type 2 diabetes. Before her diagnosis, she had not seen a doctor in 15 years because she did not have medical insurance until recently. She is very anxious about her diagnosis and doesn't understand what she needs to do to manage her condition and prevent complications. She has limited understanding of English and has difficulty with vision, but she has a large extended family, including a daughter who brought her to the office today and can act as an interpreter.

Scoring Criteria (1 Thru 4)	Excellent Evidence of Learning 4	Adequate Evidence of Learning 3	Limited Evidence of Learning 2	Unacceptable Evidence of Learning 1	Score Attempt 1	Score Attempt 2	Score Attempt 3
Demonstrates respect for individual diversity	Student demonstrates the highest level of respect for diversity when planning an appropriate education intervention	Student demonstrates mastery level of respect for diversity but does not apply the principles comprehensively	Student is developing competency in respect for diversity	Student demonstrates the main concepts of respect for diversity but does not perform them adequately			
Demonstrates empathy, active listening, and nonverbal communication skills	Student demonstrates empathy and uses restatement, reflection, and clarification when interacting with the patient. Student attends to the patient's nonverbal behaviors throughout the interview	Student demonstrates mastery level of empathy, active listening techniques, and attending to nonverbal behaviors but does not apply the principles comprehensively	Student is developing competency in demonstration of empathy, active listening techniques, and attending to nonverbal behaviors	Student demonstrates the main concepts of empathy, active listening techniques, and attending to nonverbal behaviors but does not perform them adequately			
Recognizes the importance of the patient's holistic education needs	Correctly identifies patient's diverse communication needs	Recognizes some of the patient's diverse communication needs but the approach is not comprehensive	Limited recognition of patient's diverse communication needs	Fails to identify patient's diverse communication needs			
Analyzes the situation and synthesizes a resolution	Considers all of the patient factors before reaching a solution	Identifies most of the patient factors	Limited recognition of patient factors	Fails to identify significant patient factors			
Evaluates the outcome of the intervention	Assesses the patient's understanding of the interaction	Briefly considers the patient's understanding of the interaction	Limited consideration of the patient's understanding of the interaction	Fails to evaluate the patient's understanding of the interaction			

Instructor Comments

Student Name _____ Date_____

AFFECTIVE COMPETENCY: V.A4. EXPLAIN TO A PATIENT THE RATIONALE FOR PERFORMANCE OF A PROCEDURE

Explanation: Student must achieve a minimum score of 3 in each category to achieve competency.

The linear communication model describes communication as an interactive process involving the sender of the message, the receiver, and the crucial component of feedback to confirm reception of the message. The message can be sent by a number of different methods, such as face-to-face communication, telephone, e-mail, or letter, but there is no way to confirm that the message was actually received unless the patient provides feedback about what he or she interpreted from the message. Feedback completes the communication cycle by providing a means for us to know exactly what message the patient received and therefore whether it requires clarification.

For example, one of your responsibilities as a medical assistant will be to provide patient education on the purpose of a diagnostic study. Let's say you have an elderly patient who questions the necessity of a colonoscopy procedure that was ordered by the provider. Even though you provide a detailed explanation of the procedure, as well as a handout explaining the step-by-step process, how do you really know whether the patient understands? You ask the patient to provide feedback by explaining the process back to you. As a member of the healthcare team, you must become an effective communicator. You will play a vital role in collecting and documenting patient information. If your methods of collection or recording are faulty, the quality of patient care may be seriously impaired.

Using the following case study, role-play with your partner how you would explain to a patient the rationale for performance of a procedure.

A 72-year-old patient is scheduled for her first colonoscopy. Although the physician explained the preparation for the procedure, the patient still questions whether the procedure is necessary. Demonstrate how you would deliver clear communications about the rationale for the performance of the procedure and show how you would evaluate the patient's understanding.

Scoring Criteria (1 Thru 4)	Excellent Evidence of Learning 4	Adequate Evidence of Learning 3	Limited Evidence of Learning 2	Unacceptable Evidence of Learning 1	Score Attempt 1	Score Attempt 2	Score Attempt 3
Clearly explains the rationale for the performance of the procedure.	Student demonstrates the highest level of communication skills when explaining the rationale for the performance of the procedure	Student demonstrates mastery level of the analysis of communications in providing appropriate responses/ feedback but does not apply the principles comprehensively	Student is developing competency in the analysis of communications in providing appropriate responses/ feedback	Student demonstrates the main concepts of the analysis of communications in providing appropriate responses/ feedback but does not perform them adequately			
Recognizes the importance of the patient's socioeconomic status, age, educational level, and cultural experience	Correctly identifies the patient's needs and works to clarify for the patient the rationale for the performance of the procedure	Recognizes some of the patient's needs, but the approach for explaining the rationale for the procedure is not comprehensive	Limited recognition of patient needs and does not comprehensively explain rationale of the procedure	Fails to identify patient needs and does not explain the rationale of the procedure			

Scoring Criteria (1 Thru 4)	Excellent Evidence of Learning 4	Adequate Evidence of Learning 3	Limited Evidence of Learning 2	Unacceptable Evidence of Learning 1	Score Attempt 1	Score Attempt 2	Score Attempt 3
Analyzes the situation and synthesizes a resolution	Considers all of the patient factors before reaching a solution	Identifies most of the patient factors	Limited recognition of patient factors	Fails to identify significant patient factors			
Evaluates the outcome of the intervention	Assesses the patient's understanding of the situation by gathering patient feedback	Briefly considers the patient's understanding of the situation and uses limited feedback techniques	Limited consideration of the patient's understanding of the situation	Fails to evaluate the patient's understanding of the situation and does not ask for patient feedback			

Instructor Comments:

PROCEDURE 4-1. RESPOND TO NONVERBAL COMMUNICATION

CAAHEP COMPETENCIES: V.P.1., V.P.2., V.P.3.
ABHES COMPETENCIES: 8.f.

TASK: Observe the patient and respond appropriately to nonverbal communication. Role-play with your partner the following patient scenario.

SCENARIO: Tanya Williams, 36, is a new patient with the chief complaint (CC) of intermittent abdominal pain with alternating diarrhea and constipation. Ms. Williams has experienced this discomfort for several months and appears very frustrated. You are working in the administrative side of the practice today and have to gather initial information from Ms. Williams about the history of her complaints as well as collect her insurance information and have her sign several forms. She is sitting with her arms wrapped around her abdomen, tapping her right foot on the floor and refuses to maintain eye contact. What is her nonverbal behavior telling you and how can you establish therapeutic communication with this patient?

EQUIPMENT AND SUPPLIES:
• Patient record
• Appropriate intake forms for a new patient

Standards: Complete the procedure and all critical steps in _____ minutes with a minimum score of 85% within three attempts.

Scoring: Divide the points earned by the total possible points. Failure to perform a critical step indicated by an asterisk (*), results in an unsatisfactory overall score.

Time began _____ **Time ended** _____ **Total minutes:** _____

Steps	Possible Points	Attempt 1	Attempt 2	Attempt 3
1. Greet and identify the patient by her full name and date of birth (DOB). Introduce yourself and explain your role.	10	_____	_____	_____
*2. Ask the patient the purpose of her visit and the onset, duration, and frequency of her symptoms. Pay close attention to her body language to determine whether what she is telling you is congruent with her body language.	20	_____	_____	_____
*3. Use restatement, reflection, and clarification to gather as much information as possible about the patient's CC. Make sure all medical terminology is adequately explained.	20	_____	_____	_____
*4. Speak in a pleasant, distinct manner, remembering to maintain eye contact with your patient. Remain sensitive to the diverse needs of your patient throughout the interview process.	30	_____	_____	_____
*5. Continue to observe nonverbal patient behaviors and select the appropriate verbal response to demonstrate your sensitivity to her discomfort, frustration, and anxiety.	20	_____	_____	_____

Your partner should complete the following assessment.

Did the Student:	Yes	No
Greet and identify the patient with sensitivity and respect?	_____	_____
Attend to the patient's body language?	_____	_____
Were the patient's verbal responses congruent to nonverbal behaviors?	_____	_____
If nonverbal behaviors and the verbal message were not congruent, did the medical assistant attempt to reach congruency?	_____	_____
Were all three active listening techniques used during the interview?	_____	_____
Did the medical assistant explain medical terminology?	_____	_____
Did the medical assistant display sensitivity to the diverse needs of the patient throughout the interview process?	_____	_____
Were the medical assistant's verbal responses reflective of the needs being demonstrated by the patient?	_____	_____
Did the medical assistant use clarification at the end of the interview to make sure the patient understood what was going on?	_____	_____
Did the medical assistant request patient feedback throughout the interview to make sure the patient understood questions?	_____	_____

Comments:

Points earned _____ **÷ 100 possible points = Score** _____ **% Score**

Instructor's signature _____

PROCEDURE 4-2. APPLY FEEDBACK TECHNIQUES, INCLUDING REFLECTION, RESTATEMENT, AND CLARIFICATION, TO OBTAIN PATIENT INFORMATION

Complete this procedure with another student playing the role of the patient. Choose a student about whom you know very little to make the experience more realistic. To maintain the student's privacy, he or she does not have to share any confidential information.

MAERB/CAAHEP COMPETENCIES: V.P.1., V.P.3.
ABHES COMPETENCIES: 8.f.

TASK: Use restatement, reflection, and clarification to obtain patient information and document patient care accurately.

EQUIPMENT AND SUPPLIES:
- History form or computer and electronic health record program with the patient history window opened
- Two pens if using a paper form: a red pen for recording the patient's allergies and a black pen to meet legal documentation guidelines
- Quiet, private area

Standards: Complete the procedure and all critical steps in _____ minutes with a minimum score of 85% within three attempts.

Scoring: Divide the points earned by the total possible points. Failure to perform a critical step, indicated by an asterisk (*), results in an unsatisfactory overall score.

Time began _____ **Time ended** _____ **Total minutes:** _____

Steps	Possible Points	Attempt 1	Attempt 2	Attempt 3
1. Greet and identify the patient by full name and date of birth in a pleasant manner. Introduce yourself and explain your role.	5	_____	_____	_____
2. Take the patient to a quiet, private area for the interview and explain why the information is needed.	5	_____	_____	_____
*3. Complete the history form by using therapeutic communication techniques, including restatement, reflection, and clarification. Make sure all medical terminology is adequately explained.	10	_____	_____	_____
*4. Speak in a pleasant, distinct manner, remembering to maintain eye contact with your patient.	10	_____	_____	_____
*5. Remain sensitive to the diverse needs of your patient throughout the interview process.	10	_____	_____	_____
6. State the message to your patient. Demonstrate sensitivity appropriate to the message being delivered.	5	_____	_____	_____
*7. Allow your patient to respond to the sent message. Apply active listening skills—restatement, reflection, and clarification—as needed.	10	_____	_____	_____
*8. Restate your patient's response to make sure you understand the patient's message and to give the patient the opportunity to expand on the information.	10	_____	_____	_____

Steps	Possible Points	Attempt 1	Attempt 2	Attempt 3
*9. Use reflection as appropriate to communicate your acknowledgment of the patient's feelings. Use a "feeling" word in your response to demonstrate to the patient that you are attending to his or her emotions as well as words.	10	_____	_____	_____
*10. Explain any issues that are unclear to make sure that the patient understands the meaning of each message sent. Use clarification to make sure the patient understood any medical terminology used and to summarize the information.	10	_____	_____	_____
11. Continue to communicate back and forth, using active listening techniques to make sure that your message is understood correctly.	5	_____	_____	_____
12. Analyze communications in providing appropriate responses and feedback.	5	_____	_____	_____
13. Thank the patient for sharing the information and direct him or her back to the reception area.	5	_____	_____	_____

Your partner should complete the following assessment.

Did the Student:	Yes	No
Greet and identify the patient with sensitivity and respect?	_____	_____
Attend to the patient's body language?	_____	_____
Were the patient's verbal responses congruent to nonverbal behaviors?	_____	_____
If nonverbal behaviors and the verbal message were not congruent, did the medical assistant attempt to reach congruency?	_____	_____
Were all three active listening techniques used during the interview?	_____	_____
Did the medical assistant explain medical terminology?	_____	_____
Did the medical assistant display sensitivity to the diverse needs of the patient throughout the interview process?	_____	_____
Were the medical assistant's verbal responses reflective of the needs being demonstrated by the patient?	_____	_____
Did the medical assistant use clarification at the end of the interview to make sure the patient understood what was going on?	_____	_____
Did the medical assistant explain any medical terminology used throughout the interview?	_____	_____
Did the medical assistant request patient feedback throughout the interview to make sure the patient understood questions?	_____	_____

Comments:

Points earned _____ ÷ 100 possible points = **Score** _____ **% Score**

Instructor's signature _____

5 Patient Education

Part I: Short Answers

1. The holistic model suggests that healthcare workers should take into consideration all aspects of a patient's life, including patients' _____, _____, _____, _____, and _____ needs.

2. List important guidelines for patient education.

    a. _____

    b. _____

    c. _____

    d. _____

    e. _____

    f. _____

3. Explain patient factors that influence learning.

    a. _____

    b. _____

    c. _____

    d. _____

    e. _____

    f. _____

    g. _____

4. Summarize eight approaches to language barriers.

    a. _____

    b. _____

    c. _____

    d. _____

    e. _____

    f. _____

    g. _____

    h. _____

5. One of the most important aspects of patient teaching is to be _____ and provide information about _____ patients want to know _____ patients want to know it.

6. List 10 barriers to patient learning.

a. _____

b. _____

c. _____

d. _____

e. _____

f. _____

g. _____

h. _____

i. _____

j. _____

7. Identify five guidelines for ordering educational materials.

a. _____

b. _____

c. _____

d. _____

e. _____

8. What does the role of the medical assistant educator include?

a. _____

b. _____

c. _____

d. _____

e. _____

f. _____

g. _____

h. _____

9. Effective teaching methods include use of _____ materials, DVDs/CDs, and approved _____ sites to gather information; referral to community _____ and experts; _____ demonstration of medical skills; examination of patients' records of events; and involving _____ in the education process.

10. What is a patient navigator? Describe how a medical assistant can perform this important duty in the ambulatory care setting.

_____

_____

_____

11. Describe the role of the medical assistant as a coach for patients about health maintenance, disease prevention, and their treatment plans.

_____

_____

_____

12. Based on the patient example in your text of Mr. Ignatio, a patient with newly diagnosed type 2 diabetes, use the following checklist to design and role-play a patient-centered education program.

   a. Conduct a patient assessment.
- Consider pertinent patient factors.
- Identify barriers to learning.
- Prioritize patient information.
- Determine immediate and long-term needs.
- Decide on appropriate teaching materials and methods.

      Complete _____

   b. Prepare the teaching area and assemble necessary equipment and materials.
- Use supplies and equipment the patient will use at home.
- Provide positive feedback for correct display of skills.

      Complete _____

   c. Maintain an adequate, not too fast, pace.

      Complete _____

   d. Repeatedly ask for patient feedback to confirm understanding.
- Eliminate barriers to learning.
- Address immediate learning needs.
- Use restatement, reflection, and clarification to gather patient feedback and promote understanding.

      Complete _____

   e. Summarize the material learned or the skill mastered at the end of each teaching interaction.

      Complete _____

   f. Outline a plan for the next meeting.

      Complete _____

   g. Evaluate the teaching plan.
- Was there enough time to complete the lesson?
- Was the patient physically and psychologically ready for the information?
- Were the goals for the session reached?

      Complete _____

   h. Document the teaching intervention.
- Material covered
- Patient response or level of skill performance
- Plans for next session
- Community referrals

      Complete _____

WORKPLACE APPLICATION OPTIONS

Complete one or more of these activities and, if appropriate, share your results with the class.

1. One of the roles of the medical assistant is to help patients in need of community health education or support services. To prepare for this role, collect a minimum of 25 community resources that are available in your area. Include in your directory the name of the group and the services provided; the contact person; telephone number, address, meeting times and locations; and a related website if available. Choose one of these resources and investigate the services it provides in greater detail, either by interviewing an individual who works or volunteers in the organization or by attending one of the group's sponsored meetings. Summarize your experience and share it with your classmates.

2. Samantha, a medical assistant for a family practice office, has been asked by Dr. Norberger to create patient education files for each examination room. The file should contain handouts on chronic disease, nutrition, exercise, and a healthy lifestyle. Create a list of 15 topics that should be included in this file. Why did you choose them? How may they be helpful to the doctor and the patients?

3. As Samantha begins to obtain and develop educational supplies for the patient education files, what are some guidelines she should follow as she reviews the information available? What other teaching materials should she consider using in addition to the handouts?

4. Based on what you have learned about the Health Belief Model, complete the blank spaces in the following table.

The Health Belief Model

Principles	Definition	Patient Education
Perceived susceptibility		Supply information on risk level; individual risk based on _____ _____
Perceived _____	_____ on the seriousness of the condition and its health risks	Outline the potential _____ of the disease
Perceived benefits	Patient's belief in _____	Emphasize the _____ that can occur if patient is compliant with healthcare recommendations
Perceived _____	Patient's opinion of the _____ and psychological costs of compliance	Identify _____ and work to reduce them through patient education, family outreach, and _____
	Methods developed to activate patient compliance	
Self-efficacy	Patient has the confidence to take action toward a healthier state	

5. Discuss Dr. Elisabeth Kübler-Ross's stages of grief and include in your explanation a suggestion for therapeutic interaction with a patient in each stage.

a. _____

   _____

   _____

b. _____

   _____

   _____

c. _____

   _____

   _____

d. _____

_____

_____

e. _____

_____

_____

6. Explain how the medical assistant can perform patient education for the following patients with special needs. Coach the patient appropriately considering his or her diverse cultural factors, developmental life stage, and potential communication barriers.

a. Antonio DeMendez, a 68-year-old patient, has profound hearing loss in his left ear. He needs to be taught how to take his blood pressure medication accurately.

_____

_____

_____

_____

b. Christina Wu, a 48-year-old patient, is legally blind. She is a new patient who is visiting the office for the first time and needs to complete a health history form. The physician recommends that she follow a low-sodium diet.

_____

_____

_____

_____

c. Julio Gonzales is 17 years old and has limited English skills. He is scheduled for diagnostic testing at the hospital and must be taught how to prepare for the studies.

_____

_____

_____

_____

7. For the following scenarios, write "Yes" on the line if the medical assistant's actions are acceptable practice according to Health Insurance Portability and Accountability Act (HIPAA) guidelines or "No" if they are not acceptable.

_____ The mother of a 19-year-old patient, Sue Collins, calls the office. Even though the mother is not listed as Sue's personal health information (PHI), Taylor answers her questions about Sue's illness.

_____ The patient requests that only her husband receive information about her health status. Taylor receives a call from the patient's adult daughter, who insists on learning her mother's diagnosis. Taylor feels bad for the daughter and answers her questions.

INTERNET ACTIVITY OPTIONS

Complete this activity and, if appropriate, share your results with the class.

1. Visit the National Institutes of Health (NIH) Health Topics link at http://www.nlm.nih.gov/medlineplus/healthtopics.html. Click on any of the topics you find interesting. Do you think this site would be a good patient education choice for individuals who have access to the Internet?

1. Mary Ann has recently been diagnosed with hypercholesterolemia. As Taylor is discussing diet and exercise recommendations, Mary Ann replies that she doesn't think cholesterol is something she should be concerned about, and what with working two jobs, she is forced to dine out and eat "on the run" most days. What type of patient barriers will Taylor need to overcome? What type of patient education material should Taylor provide? Document the patient education intervention.

   _____

   _____

   _____

   _____

2. Describe how the patient's chronologic age and developmental age result in the need to adapt the teaching plan for the following patients. What changes will you make to the methods of delivery? Are any learning barriers present that must be overcome? What types of patient information will you provide to each person? Document the patient education intervention.

   a. A 74-year-old woman was recently diagnosed with type 2 diabetes. Before her diagnosis, she had not seen a doctor in 20 years. She loves to cook for her large family but complains of difficulty reading recipes because the diabetes has resulted in diabetic retinopathy.

   _____

   _____

   _____

   _____

   b. An 11-year-old boy was recently diagnosed with type 1 diabetes. He loves to play sports and is very active. His father complains that he plays so much that getting him to eat properly is difficult. The boy is afraid of needles, and the doctor has ordered him to begin using insulin and routinely checking his blood glucose levels with a glucometer.

   _____

   _____

   _____

   _____

PROCEDURE 5-1. DEVELOP A LIST OF COMMUNITY RESOURCES FOR PATIENTS' HEALTHCARE NEEDS; ALSO, FACILITATE REFERRALS IN THE ROLE OF PATIENT NAVIGATOR

CAAHEP COMPETENCIES: V.P.9., V.P.10.
ABHES COMPETENCIES: 5.c., 9.i.

TASK: Develop a list of community resources and perform the role of the patient navigator by referring patients to resources

One of the roles of the medical assistant is to help patients in need of community health education or support services. To prepare for this role, collect a minimum of 25 community resources such as support groups, educational workshops, dietary assistance, national organizations, medical equipment suppliers, and so forth, that are available in your area. Include in your directory the name of the group and the services provided; the contact person; telephone number, address, meeting times and locations; and a related website. As a patient navigator, apply what you have learned about community resources to assist the patient in the following case study.

SCENARIO: Mr. Tomas Garcia was admitted to the hospital last week for an acute myocardial infarction (MI). Mr. Garcia is 54 years old, is overweight, smokes two packs of cigarettes a day, eats fast food almost daily, has a family history of heart disease, and works as a carpenter. The provider recommends he lose weight, follow a high-fiber, reduced saturated-fat diet, and quit smoking. What community resources might help educate and support Mr. Garcia with these complex lifestyle changes?

EQUIPMENT AND SUPPLIES:
- Patient's health record
- Educational handouts
- Computer with Internet connection and printer
- Quiet, private area

Standards: Complete the procedure and all critical steps in _____ minutes with a minimum score of 85% within three attempts.

Scoring: Divide the points earned by the total possible points. Failure to perform a critical step, indicated by an asterisk (*), results in an unsatisfactory overall score.

Time began _____ Time ended _____ Total minutes: _____

Steps	Possible Points	Attempt 1	Attempt 2	Attempt 3
1. Greet and identify the patient in a pleasant manner. Introduce yourself and explain your role.	5	_____	_____	_____
2. Take the patient to a quiet, private area. Ideally, the room has a computer with Internet access and access to a printer so that you can conduct an individualized search for community resources.	5	_____	_____	_____
*3. Assess Mr. Garcia's needs and identify factors that may limit his ability to learn and implement lifestyle changes. Use restatement, reflection, and clarification to verify the information.	25	_____	_____	_____
4. Speak in a pleasant, distinct manner, remembering to maintain eye contact with your patient.	10	_____	_____	_____
*5. Remain sensitive to the diverse needs of your patient throughout the interview process, including his health, family, and diet histories and the recommendations of the provider.	15	_____	_____	_____

Steps	Possible Points	Attempt 1	Attempt 2	Attempt 3
*6. Provide Mr. Garcia with appropriate handouts and conduct an online search of provider-approved community resources that might be of benefit. Print out this information or e-mail it to the patient for future use.	20	_____	_____	_____
*7. Use clarification and feedback methods to make sure the patient does not have any questions.	15	_____	_____	_____
8. Document the patient education intervention in the health record.	5	_____	_____	_____

Comments:

Points earned _____ ÷ 100 possible points = **Score** _____ **% Score**

Instructor's signature _____

PROCEDURE 5-2. COACH PATIENTS IN HEALTH MAINTENANCE, DISEASE PREVENTION, AND FOLLOWING THE TREATMENT PLAN

CAAHEP COMPETENCIES: V.P.4., V.A.3.
ABHES COMPETENCIES: 5.e., 9.j.

TASK: Coach patients about health maintenance, disease prevention, and the treatment plan while appropriately considering individual patient factors

SCENARIO: Carmen Barone is a 78-year-old patient who was recently diagnosed with type 2 diabetes. Before her diagnosis, she had not seen a doctor in 20 years. She is overweight, has a family history of diabetes, has hearing aids but rarely uses them, and loves to cook for her large Italian family. She has difficulty reading and is at risk for developing foot ulcers because of diabetic complications. One of the goals of the patient education intervention is to teach Mrs. Barone how to use a glucometer so she can monitor her blood glucose levels at home.

EQUIPMENT AND SUPPLIES:
• Patent health record
• Educational handouts and/or access to online resources that can be printed
• Quiet, private area

Standards: Complete the procedure and all critical steps in _____ minutes with a minimum score of 85% within three attempts.

Scoring: Divide the points earned by the total possible points. Failure to perform a critical step, indicated by an asterisk (*), results in an unsatisfactory overall score.

Time began _____ Time ended _____ Total minutes: _____

Steps	Possible Points	Attempt 1	Attempt 2	Attempt 3
1. Greet and identify the patient in a pleasant manner. Introduce yourself and explain your role.	5	_____	_____	_____
2. Take the patient to a quiet, private area. Ideally, the room has a computer with Internet access and access to a printer so that you can conduct an individualized search for education materials and community resources.	5	_____	_____	_____
*3. Identify factors that may limit the patient's ability to learn and implement lifestyle changes.	20	_____	_____	_____
*4. Prioritize the patient information and determine the patient's immediate and long-term needs.	10	_____	_____	_____
*5. Prepare the teaching area and assemble necessary equipment and materials, making sure to use the same supplies and equipment the patient will use at home.	10	_____	_____	_____
*6. Use restatement, reflection, and clarification to promote understanding throughout the teaching intervention.	10	_____	_____	_____
*7. Remain sensitive to the diverse needs of your patient throughout the interview process, including cultural background and problems with vision and hearing.	10	_____	_____	_____

20. An individual who is prone to engage in lawsuits is considered _____.

21. _____ is a type of negligence in which a medical professional fails to provide the standard of care, causing harm to another.

22. An individual who is assigned by the court to be legally responsible for protecting the well-being and interests of a ward is identified as a(n) _____.

23. A harmful, false statement made about another person identified legally as an oral defamation or insult is called _____.

24. Information that is significant and demonstrates bearing on the matter at hand is considered _____.

25. An individual who acts with wisdom when managing practical affairs is considered _____.

26. _____ are businesses that receive healthcare transactions from healthcare providers, translate the data from a given format into one acceptable to the intended payor, and forward the processed transaction to designated payors; this includes billing services, community health information systems, and private network providers or "value-added" networks that facilitate electronic data interchanges.

27. A(n) _____ contract is one that is assumed to exist. For example, if a patient is being seen by a provider for the first time, it is assumed that the patient will provide a comprehensive and accurate health history and that the provider will diagnose and treat the patient in good faith to the best of his or her ability.

28. A _____ of contract occurs if there is a failure to perform any term of a contract, written or oral, without a legitimate legal excuse.

29. Civil law involves cases that are brought to court by _____.

30. Criminal law involves a crime against the _____ or _____.

SKILLS AND CONCEPTS

1. What are the four elements that are essential to a valid legal contract?

   a. _____

   b. _____

   c. _____

   d. _____

2. The physician–patient relationship is generally held by courts to be a contractual relationship that is the result of three steps. What are they?

   a. _____

   b. _____

   c. _____

3. If the patient does not pay for the services rendered by the provider, does this negate the physician–patient contract?

   _____

   _____

   _____

4. If a provider decides to terminate the care agreement for a patient, what methods should be followed and what details should be included in a letter of notification?

_____

_____

_____

5. How can the medical assistant help protect the provider against a lawsuit for abandonment?

_____

_____

_____

6. Describe the difference between a misdemeanor and a felony.

_____

_____

_____

7. Explain the details of a defamation case under tort law.

_____

_____

_____

8. Explain the difference between a deposition and an interrogatory.

_____

_____

_____

9. List three of the five ways to determine whether a subpoena is valid.

a. _____

b. _____

c. _____

10. Explain the importance of discovery in a medical professional liability case.

_____

_____

_____

11. Explain the difference between mediation and arbitration.

_____

_____

_____

12. Why are alternative dispute resolutions important tools in resolving a medical malpractice case?

_____

_____

_____

13. Define medical malpractice and negligence.

_____

_____

_____

14. List the three general classifications of medical professional negligence.

a. _____

b. _____

c. _____

15. What is contributory negligence?

_____

_____

_____

16. What four elements must be present in a medical professional liability case before negligence can be proven?

a. _____

b. _____

c. _____

d. _____

17. Explain the five types of damages that are common in tort cases.

a. _____

b. _____

c. _____

d. _____

e. _____

18. Summarize five features that should be included in a healthcare facility's risk management practices.

a. _____

b. _____

c. _____

d. _____

e. _____

19. Explain the doctrine of *respondeat superior* and its significance in medical assistant practice.

_____

_____

_____

20. The administrative medical assistant may be involved in either researching or renewing insurance policies for their employers. Explain the three types of insurance discussed in the chapter.

a. _____

b. _____

c. _____

21. What are the differences among implied consent, expressed consent, and informed consent?

_____

_____

_____

22. An exception to the need for parental consent is if the individual is an emancipated minor. Explain how an individual under the age of 18 might be eligible for emancipation.

_____

_____

_____

23. Explain what is meant when an individual is declared incompetent and how it can legally be decided.

_____

_____

_____

24. What is the Patient Self-Determination Act? In your description include a discussion about advance directives and a medical durable power of attorney.

_____

_____

_____

25. List the provisions of the Uniform Anatomical Gift Act.

_____

_____

_____

26. Summarize how the ADAA and GINA legislation support and protect the rights of affected individuals in our society.

_____

_____

_____

27. Summarize five important features of the Health Insurance Portability and Accountability Act (HIPAA) Privacy Rule.

a. _____

b. _____

c. _____

d. _____

e. _____

28. Why is the HITECH Act a significant piece of legislation for healthcare facilities?

_____

_____

_____

29. The Affordable Care Act enacted major health insurance reforms and was designed to enhance the quality of care for all Americans. Summarize five important features that were put into place immediately after the law was passed in 2010.

a. _____

b. _____

c. _____

d. _____

e. _____

30. Describe compliance with public health statutes regarding reporting communicable diseases; abuse, neglect, and exploitation; and wounds of violence.

_____

_____

_____

_____

31. Define the following terms/abbreviations that are associated with HIPAA.

a. NPP _____

b. Covered entities _____

c. PHI _____

d. Covered transactions _____

e. State's preemption of HIPAA regulations _____

f. Minimum necessary standard _____

g. TPO _____

32. Explain what is meant by a limited data set and how this HIPAA rule may affect medical assistants.

_____

_____

_____

33. The HIPAA Security Rule (SR) covers the use and transmission of electronic Protected Health Information (ePHI). Summarize the safeguards for protection of ePHI.

_____

_____

_____

34. Define the term *locum tenens* and explain how it affects medical assistants in the professional workplace.

_____

_____

_____

35. Summarize the Patient's Bill of Rights.

_____

_____

_____

36. Compare criminal and civil law as they apply to the practicing medical assistant.

_____

_____

_____

37. Define the following:

a. Statute of limitations

_____

_____

_____

b. Good Samaritan Act(s)

_____

_____

c. Risk management

_____

_____

d. Mature minor

_____

_____

CASE STUDY

Teresa Guelerro is a 58-year-old patient diagnosed with terminal breast cancer. She has been reading about advance directives but she doesn't understand the meaning of some of the terminology on the form. How can the medical assistant help Mrs. Guelerro? In your answer include the meaning of the typical categories of treatment listed on an advance directive and suggest some community or online resources that might help her create her own document.

_____

_____

_____

_____

_____

53

WORKPLACE APPLICATIONS

Complete one or more of these activities and share your results with the class, if appropriate.

1. HIPAA regulations protect the privacy of a patient's health information. Summarize what you learned about HIPAA and apply it to practices that should be followed in the workplace.

_____

_____

_____

_____

_____

2. Summarize how the medical assistant can apply the Patient's Bill of Rights to everyday practice in the healthcare setting.

_____

_____

_____

_____

_____

3. The Four Ds of Negligence and Damages

   a. A patient was given the wrong medication. No adverse effects occurred. Which of the four Ds is missing? Why does this affect the possibility of a lawsuit?

   _____

   _____

   _____

   _____

   _____

   b. A patient is treated for low back pain caused by a fall at the local mall. The patient sues the physician, because the pain is unresolved. Which of the four Ds would be the most difficult for the patient's attorney to prove? Why?

   _____

   _____

   _____

   _____

   _____

INTERNET ACTIVITIES

1. Research the American Bar Association's Consumer's Toolkit for Health Care Advance Planning at www .americanbar.org/groups/law_aging/resources/health_care_decision_making/consumer_s_toolkit_for_health_care _advance_planning.html. Could this be a helpful resource for patients attempting to develop an advance directive?

2. Research the Affordable Care Act online. Do you or anyone you know have personal experience with the insurance marketplace? What are the advantages and disadvantages of the law? Discuss your findings with the class.

Student Name _____ Date_____

AFFECTIVE COMPETENCIES: X.A1. DEMONSTRATE SENSITIVITY TO PATIENT RIGHTS

Explanation: Student must achieve a minimum score of 3 in each category to achieve competency.

Risk management strategies are those steps employed by all members of the healthcare team to prevent patients from bringing suit against the physician and/or practice. Medical assistants play an important role in preventing malpractice suits by consistently applying risk management strategies. Risk management behaviors and actions are designed to identify, contain, reduce, or eliminate the potential for patient harm and ultimately financial loss to the practice. The facility's policies and procedures are designed to manage risk and prevent situations that could result in harm to people or property for which the facility could be held liable. Therefore all employees must strictly follow the policies and procedures adopted by their employers. In addition, the medical assistant should always practice within the legal boundaries of the state of residence.

Medical liability often starts with a patient who is not happy with the type of service received in the facility and/or who has not developed a personal relationship with care providers. Therefore the first step in risk management is therapeutic communications. Other important factors include consistently performing respectful patient care, demonstrating your concern for patients, incorporating patients into the plan of care as active participants in their own health, providing research-based materials about patient conditions and suggesting reputable websites for additional information, encouraging patients to ask questions and clarify treatment plans, and meticulous documentation of all patient interactions so there is a comprehensive and detailed written record of patient care.

The Patient's Bill of Rights should be kept in mind each time the medical assistant interacts with a patient. For example, you should explain procedures to patients and make sure they understand treatments. Printed information about the facility should contain details about how and where a patient can make a complaint about the care received. Policies and procedures should honor the provisions of the Patient's Bill of Rights in everyday practice in the healthcare setting.

Using the following case study, role-play with your partner how you would demonstrate sensitivity to patient rights.

You are employed as a clinical medical assistant in a large multiphysician cardiology practice. A patient just told you that she is no longer going to take her cardiac medication as prescribed by the physician. Does the patient have the right to refuse treatment? Role-play how you will inform the physician of the patient's decision.

Scoring Criteria (1 thru 4)	Excellent Evidence of Learning 4	Adequate Evidence of Learning 3	Limited Evidence of Learning 2	Unacceptable Evidence of Learning 1	Score Attempt 1	Score Attempt 2	Score Attempt 3
Demonstrates sensitivity to patient rights	Student demonstrates the highest level of sensitivity to patient rights by performing respectful patient care and encouraging patients to ask questions and clarify treatment plans	Student demonstrates mastery level of sensitivity to patient rights but does not encourage the patient to ask questions to clarify the treatment plan	Student is developing competency in sensitivity to patient rights but does not encourage the patient to ask questions to clarify the treatment plan	Student does not demonstrate sensitivity to patient rights			

Chapter **6** **Medicine and Law**

Scoring Criteria (1 thru 4)	Excellent Evidence of Learning 4	Adequate Evidence of Learning 3	Limited Evidence of Learning 2	Unacceptable Evidence of Learning 1	Score Attempt 1	Score Attempt 2	Score Attempt 3
Communicates effectively with the physician regarding the patient's decision not to follow the treatment plan	Student uses active listening and therapeutic communications to professionally communicate with the physician the patient's decision not to follow the treatment plan	Student communicates the patient's decision to the physician but does not use comprehensive active listening skills to deliver the message	Limited use of effective communication skills with the physician regarding the patient's decision not to follow the treatment plan	Student fails to communicate effectively with the physician the patient's decision not to follow the treatment plan			

Instructor Comments:

PROCEDURE 6-1. APPLY THE PATIENTS' BILL OF RIGHTS IN CHOICE OF TREATMENT, CONSENT FOR TREATMENT, AND REFUSAL OF TREATMENT

CAAHEP COMPETENCY: X.P.4.
ABHES COMPETENCY: 4.g.

TASK: Ensure that the patient's rights are honored in the daily procedures performed and policies enacted in the ambulatory healthcare setting.

SCENARIO: Role-play with a partner the following case study that requires the application of the Patient's Bill of Rights as it pertains to treatment choices, consent for treatment, and refusal of treatment.

Dr. Patrick recommends that Mr. Tim Shields start taking Rituxan (rituximab) for non–Hodgkin's lymphoma (NHL). She provides informed consent to Mr. Shields about the risks of Rituxan, including the possibility of a serious allergic reaction, severe skin and mouth reactions, and an increased risk of serious or life-threatening complications if the patient has hepatitis B. Dr. Patrick also explains that this is the best treatment option for Mr. Shields. There are other possible treatment options, but Rituxan is the recommended drug of choice for treatment of NHL.

Mr. Shields states that he understands the information. He is hesitant to give informed consent, however, because he has a history of hepatitis B and is concerned about the serious side effects from the drug. Mr. Shields opts to refuse the Rituxan treatment. Based on your knowledge of the Patient's Bill of Rights, has Dr. Patrick complied with the provider part of the agreement? Does Mr. Shields have the right to refuse the recommended medication? If he does refuse, is it important that his refusal of recommended treatment be documented in his health record? How can the medical assistant help both the provider and patient in this situation?

EQUIPMENT AND SUPPLIES:
- Copy of the Patients' Bill of Rights
- Notice of Privacy Practices form

Standards: Complete the procedure and all critical steps in _____ minutes with a minimum score of 85% within three attempts.

Scoring: Divide the points earned by the total possible points. Failure to perform a critical step, indicated by an asterisk (*), results in an unsatisfactory overall score.

Time began _____ Time ended _____ Total minutes: _____

Steps	Possible Points	Attempt 1	Attempt 2	Attempt 3
1. Review the Patients' Bill of Rights.	10	_____	_____	_____
*2. The patient has the right to receive information about his or her health plan, professionals, facilities, and personal care. Role-play the information the physician gave Mr. Shields about his treatment choices.	10	_____	_____	_____
*3. The patient has the right to choose a healthcare provider, but patients may have restrictions on those choices according to their insurance plan. Role-play that Dr. Patrick's services are covered by Mr. Shields's insurance.	10	_____	_____	_____
*4. The patient has the right to receive referral to emergency facilities and for emergency treatment in the office. Role-play a discussion with Mr. Shields about how he can contact the facility or Dr. Patrick if he has a medical emergency.	10	_____	_____	_____

Steps	Possible Points	Attempt 1	Attempt 2	Attempt 3
*5. The patient has the right to know all treatment options and to participate in decisions about care. Role-play the information that Dr. Patrick gave Mr. Shields about his care and treatment choices.	10	_____	_____	_____
*6. The patient has the right to considerate, respectful, and nondiscriminatory care by all healthcare staff. Role-play respectful care toward Mr. Shields.	10	_____	_____	_____
*7. Patients have the right to review their records and to expect confidential treatment of their healthcare information. Review methods of enforcing patient confidentiality in the facility. Role-play the patient completing a patient's Notice of Privacy Practices form. Role-play a scenario in which Mr. Shields's girlfriend calls and asks you to tell her what Dr. Patrick suggested for treatment. She is not identified on the patient's Notice of Privacy Practices form. Can you give her that information?	10	_____	_____	_____
*8. The patient has the right to a fair and objective review of complaints. During your interaction with Mr. Shields, he complains about how long he had to wait for his appointment and that the receptionist was rude. Role-play how you should manage Mr. Shields's complaints.	10	_____	_____	_____
*9. The patient has the responsibility to be involved in care. Mr. Shields has opted to refuse medical treatment and try a homeopathic approach to treatment of his cancer. Role-play your interaction with Mr. Shields about follow-up with Dr. Patrick.	10	_____	_____	_____
*10. Demonstrate sensitivity to patients' rights through empathy, use of therapeutic communication, and respect for individual diversity.	10	_____	_____	_____

Comments:

Points earned _____ ÷ 100 possible points = **Score** _____ **% Score**

Instructor's signature _____

Name _____ Date _____ Score _____

PROCEDURE 6-2. APPLY HIPAA RULES ON PRIVACY AND RELEASE OF INFORMATION AND REPORT ILLEGAL ACTIVITY IN THE HEALTHCARE SETTING

CAAHEP COMPETENCIES: X.P.2., X.P.6.
ABHES COMPETENCIES: 4.b., 4.f.

TASK: Be aware of HIPAA privacy and release of information rules and apply them in the ambulatory care center.

Although not specifically required by HIPAA, practices may want to use a routine patient consent form that specifies methods by which a patient agrees to let the practice notify the patient of routine treatment, payment, and healthcare operations (TPO).

SCENARIO: You recently graduated from a CAAHEP-accredited medical assisting program and just passed the certification examination to earn the CMA (AAMA) credential. You learned a great deal about HIPAA applications in your medical assisting program and are confident that you can apply these regulations in the family practice where you are working. A patient comes to the office today very upset because a message about her laboratory test results was left on her home answering machine, even though she specifically requested in her disclosure consent form that messages only be left on her cell phone. Her mother then called the facility and requested information about her diagnosis. How should this situation be handled? The office manager does nothing to correct this error. Can the patient and/or the medical assistant report this infraction of the Privacy Rule to the Office for Civil Rights (OCR)? How can this be done? The patient decides to switch physicians because of her dissatisfaction with the management of her personal health information. Role-play the application of HIPAA privacy and release of information rules in this case.

EQUIPMENT AND SUPPLIES:
• Computer with Internet access
• Copy of facility PHI consent form
• Notice of Privacy Practices form
• Authorization for Release of Medical Records

Standards: Complete the procedure and all critical steps in _____ minutes with a minimum score of 85% within three attempts.

Scoring: Divide the points earned by the total possible points. Failure to perform a critical step, indicated by an asterisk (*), results in an unsatisfactory overall score.

Time began _____ **Time ended** _____ **Total minutes:** _____

Steps	Possible Points	Attempt 1	Attempt 2	Attempt 3
1. Consistently review and apply HIPAA regulations that apply to the facility.	5	_____	_____	_____
*2. Identify the ramifications of noncompliance with HIPAA's Privacy Rule. Role-play the scenario presented. Did the facility comply with the Privacy Rule and the proper release of information?	15	_____	_____	_____
*3. Routinely apply Privacy Rule regulations to all operations in the medical office. Role-play how the patient's confidentiality and privacy should have been maintained.	15	_____	_____	_____
*4. Follow patient-directed methods of contact when TPO information must be left on an answering machine, mailed, or e-mailed. Role-play the correct way of contacting the patient about personal health information.	15	_____	_____	_____

59

Steps	Possible Points	Attempt 1	Attempt 2	Attempt 3
*5. Always follow office policy when performing any action that is covered under HIPAA rules.	10	_____	_____	_____
*6. Report HIPAA violations as you see fit to the appropriate supervisor in the medical facility. Role-play the methods for reporting HIPAA violations in the facility.	15	_____	_____	_____
*7. If appropriate, report HIPAA violations to the Office for Civil Rights at the Department of Health and Human Services (*https://ocrportal.hhs.gov/ocr/cp/wizard_cp.jsf*) or file a complaint in writing by mail, fax, or e-mail. Role-play how you could assist the patient in reporting a privacy violation.	15	_____	_____	_____
8. The patient decides to switch providers because of her dissatisfaction with the care provided in the facility. Role-play the completion of an Authorization for Release of Medical Records form.	5	_____	_____	_____
9. Demonstrate sensitivity to patients' rights through empathy, use of therapeutic communication, and respect for individual diversity.	5	_____	_____	_____

Comments:

Points earned _____ ÷ 100 possible points = **Score** _____ **% Score**

Instructor's signature _____

Name: _____

WORK PRODUCT 6-1. PATIENT HIPAA ACKNOWLEDGMENT

Corresponds to PROCEDURE 6-1

CAAHEP COMPETENCY: X.P.4.
ABHES COMPETENCY: 4.g.

PATIENT HIPAA ACKNOWLEDGEMENT

I. **Acknowledgement of Practice's *Notice of Privacy Practices*:**

By subscribing my name below, I acknowledge that I was provided a copy of the Notice of Privacy Practices and that I have read (or had the opportunity to read if I so chose) and understand the Notice of Privacy Practices and agree to its terms.

_____ _____ _____
Name of Patient/Date of Birth   Signature of Patient/Parent/Guardian   Date

II. **Designation of Certain Relatives, Close Friends, and other Caregivers as my Personal Representative:**

I agree that the practice may disclose certain pieces of my health information to a Personal Representative of my choosing, since such person is involved with my healthcare or payment relating to my healthcare. In that case, the Physician Practice will disclose only information that is directly relevant to the person's involvement with my healthcare or payment relating to my health care.

Print Name: _____ Last four digits of SSN or other identifier: _____

Print Name: _____ Last four digits of SSN or other identifier: _____

Print Name: _____ Last four digits of SSN or other identifier: _____

III. **Request to Receive Confidential Communications by Alternative Means:**

As provided by Privacy Rule Section 164.522(b), I hereby request that the Practice make all communications to me by the alternative means that I have listed below.

Home or Cell Telephone Number: **Written Communication Address:**

_____   _____

____ OK to leave message with detailed information   ____ OK to mail to address listed above
____ Leave message with call back numbers only   ____ E-mail me at:_____

Work Telephone Number: **E-mail Communication:**

_____   _____

____ OK to leave message with detailed information   ____ OK to text at the number listed above
____ Leave message with call back numbers only   ____ E-mail me at:_____

Other:_____

IV. **The following person(s) <u>are not authorized</u> to receive my Patient Health Information (PHI):**

Print Name:_____   Print Name:_____

Print Name:_____   Print Name:_____

Chapter **6** **Medicine and Law**

V. **The HIPAA Privacy rule requires healthcare providers to take reasonable steps to limit the use** or disclosure of, and requests for PHI. I understand that this accounting will not reflect disclosures that are made in the course of the Practice's ordinary health care activities related to providing patient treatment, obtaining payment for its services or its internal operations. Also, the Practice does not have to account for disclosures for which I have executed an Authorization permitting disclosures of my PHI.

Date of disclosure request	Disclosed to whom: address/e-mail	Description of disclosure	Purpose of disclosure	Dates of Service of disclosure	Person completing request	Date completed

1. The above authorizations are voluntary and I may refuse to agree to their terms without affecting any of my rights to receive healthcare at the Practice.

2. These Authorizations may be revoked at any time by notifying the Practice in writing at the Practice's mailing address marked to the attention of "HIPAA Compliance Officer."

3. The revocation of this authorization will not have any effect on disclosures occurring prior to the execution of any revocation.

4. I may see and copy the information described in this form, if I ask for it, and I will get a copy of this form after I sign it.

5. This form was completely filled in before I signed it and I acknowledge that all of my questions were answered to my satisfaction, that I fully understand this authorization form, and have received an executed copy.

6. This authorization is valid as of the date I have signed below and shall remain valid until changed or revoked.

_____   _____   _____
Name of Patient (Printed)   Signature of Patient   Date

WORK PRODUCT 6-2. PATIENT HIPAA ACKNOWLEDGMENT

Corresponds to PROCEDURE 6-2

CAAHEP COMPETENCIES: X.P.2., X.P.6.
ABHES COMPETENCIES: 4.b., 4.f.

PATIENT HIPAA ACKNOWLEDGEMENT

I.   Acknowledgement of Practice's *Notice of Privacy Practices*:

By subscribing my name below, I acknowledge that I was provided a copy of the Notice of Privacy Practices and that I have read (or had the opportunity to read if I so chose) and understand the Notice of Privacy Practices and agree to its terms.

_____	_____	_____
Name of Patient/Date of Birth	Signature of Patient/Parent/Guardian	Date

II.   Designation of Certain Relatives, Close Friends, and other Caregivers as my Personal Representative:

I agree that the practice may disclose certain pieces of my health information to a Personal Representative of my choosing, since such person is involved with my healthcare or payment relating to my healthcare. In that case, the Physician Practice will disclose only information that is directly relevant to the person's involvement with my healthcare or payment relating to my health care.

Print Name: _____ Last four digits of SSN or other identifier: _____

Print Name: _____ Last four digits of SSN or other identifier: _____

Print Name: _____ Last four digits of SSN or other identifier: _____

III. Request to Receive Confidential Communications by Alternative Means:

As provided by Privacy Rule Section 164.522(b), I hereby request that the Practice make all communications to me by the alternative means that I have listed below.

Home or Cell Telephone Number: **Written Communication Address:**

_____   _____

____ OK to leave message with detailed information   ____ OK to mail to address listed above
____ Leave message with call back numbers only   ____ E-mail me at:_____

Work Telephone Number: **E-mail Communication:**

_____   _____

____ OK to leave message with detailed information   ____ OK to text at the number listed above
____ Leave message with call back numbers only   ____ E-mail me at:_____

Other:_____

IV.   The following person(s) <u>are not authorized</u> to receive my Patient Health Information (PHI):

Print Name: _____   Print Name: _____

Print Name: _____   Print Name: _____

Chapter **6**   Medicine and Law

V. **The HIPAA Privacy rule requires healthcare providers to take reasonable steps to limit the use** or disclosure of, and requests for PHI. I understand that this accounting will not reflect disclosures that are made in the course of the Practice's ordinary health care activities related to providing patient treatment, obtaining payment for its services or its internal operations. Also, the Practice does not have to account for disclosures for which I have executed an Authorization permitting disclosures of my PHI.

Date of disclosure request	Disclosed to whom: address/e-mail	Description of disclosure	Purpose of disclosure	Dates of Service of disclosure	Person completing request	Date completed

1. The above authorizations are voluntary and I may refuse to agree to their terms without affecting any of my rights to receive healthcare at the Practice.

2. These Authorizations may be revoked at any time by notifying the Practice in writing at the Practice's mailing address marked to the attention of "HIPAA Compliance Officer."

3. The revocation of this authorization will not have any effect on disclosures occurring prior to the execution of any revocation.

4. I may see and copy the information described in this form, if I ask for it, and I will get a copy of this form after I sign it.

5. This form was completely filled in before I signed it and I acknowledge that all of my questions were answered to my satisfaction, that I fully understand this authorization form, and have received an executed copy.

6. This authorization is valid as of the date I have signed below and shall remain valid until changed or revoked.

_____   _____   _____

Name of Patient (Printed)   Signature of Patient   Date

WORK PRODUCT 6-3. PATIENT CONSENT FOR USE AND DISCLOSURE OF PROTECTED HEALTH INFORMATION

Kennedy Family Practice
414 Jacksonia St., Armandale, VA. 26004

Patient Consent for Use and Disclosure
of Protected Health Information

I hereby give my consent for Kennedy Family Practice to use and disclose protected health information (PHI) about me to carry out treatment, payment and health care operations (TPO).

I have the right to review the Notice of Privacy Practices prior to signing this consent. Kennedy Family Practice reserves the right to revise its Notice of Privacy Practices at any time. A revised Notice of Privacy Practices may be obtained by forwarding a written request to Sophia Viero, 414 Jacksonia St., Armandale, VA. 26004.

With this consent, a representative of Kennedy Family Practice may call my home or other alternative location and leave a message on voice mail or in person; may e-mail me on my approved email site; and/or may mail to my home or other alternative location any items that assist the practice in carrying out TPO such as appointment reminders, insurance items, and any calls pertaining to my clinical care, including laboratory test results.

I have the right to request that Kennedy Family Practice restrict how it uses or discloses my PHI to carry out TPO. By signing this form, I am consenting to allow Kennedy Family Practice to use and disclose my PHI to carry out TPO.

I may revoke my consent in writing; however, previous disclosures are considered valid based on my prior consent.

_____
Signature of Patient or Legal Guardian

_____   _____
Print Patient's Name   Date

_____   _____
Patient Approved Telephone number   Patient Approved Email address

WORK PRODUCT 6-4. AUTHORIZATION FOR RELEASE OF MEDICAL RECORDS

Authorization for Release of Medical Records

Kennedy Family Practice
414 Jacksonia St., Armandale, VA. 26004

Name of Patient:
_____

Date of Birth: _____Phone: _____

The information being disclosed may include: HIV/AIDS, Drug/Alcohol Abuse & Mental Health data. This document authorizes release of information entered into my medical record prior to or within 12 months after the date of my signature.

Release Medical Records To:
_____

(Name of Authorized Person, Agency, Institution or other)
_____

Street Address
_____

City   State   Zip Code

Format in which you would like to release or receive medical records information:

Medical Record on Paper   Faxed Medical Record

Medical Records via Internet

Reason for Request:
_____
_____
_____

Please provide the **type(s) of medical records** information requested:
_____
_____
_____

I hereby release the provider of said records from any legal responsibility or liability in connection with the release of the records indicated herein.

_____

Signature of Patient or Representative   Date

_____

Relationship if signed by other than Patient

There could be an associated fee incurred by you for medical records requests. The current fees are:
Pages 1-5 No Charge
Pages 6-20 $1.44 per page
Pages 21-60 $1.06 per page
Pages 61-end $0.35 per page
Microfilm/Microfiche $2.12 per page
Plus applicable postage and tax

Chapter **6** Medicine and Law

7 Medicine and Ethics

Fill in the blanks with the correct vocabulary terms from this chapter.

1. Melissa believes that one of her roles as a medical assistant is to be a patient _____, a person who pleads and defends the cause of another.

2. Jill understands that the _____ of her actions while she is at work could affect whether a patient complies with the physician's instructions.

3. Kristy considers being friendly toward the patients in the clinic as her _____ and a vital part of her job performance.

4. When a person has breached an ethical standard, _____ may be necessary to atone for the action.

Define the following:

1. Sociologic _____

2. Public domain _____

3. Procurement _____

4. Upcoding _____

SKILLS AND CONCEPTS

1. What is the difference between ethics and morals?

   _____

   _____

   _____

2. What do you value most in life? What is important to you? What influences you to act in a certain way? Make a list of five things you value the most and share them with the class. Try to determine why you feel so strongly about those particular things.

   _____

   _____

   _____

3. Honestly evaluate your personal biases. What do you find unacceptable in people? Do you prejudge an individual based on his or her affiliation with a particular group or because of a certain lifestyle decision? Do these biases create barriers to ethical care? If so, how can you get beyond these barriers?

   _____

   _____

   _____

4. What is the difference between personal and professional ethics?

_____

_____

_____

5. Discuss the effect that personal morals and values have on professional performance.

_____

_____

_____

6. Summarize the ethical concepts included in the American Association of Medical Assistants (AAMA) Code of Ethics.

_____

_____

_____

7. How might the AAMA Medical Assisting Creed help guide a medical assistant who is facing complex ethical and moral issues in the course of his or her work?

_____

_____

_____

8. If you plan to seek the CMA (AAMA) credential you will be expected to follow a Code of Conduct for medical assistants. The Code includes:

_____

_____

_____

9. Explain the four types of ethical duties related to the medical profession.

a. _____

b. _____

c. _____

d. _____

10. List and define the four types of ethical problems that individuals in healthcare may face.

a. _____

b. _____

c. _____

d. _____

11. Summarize the five steps of ethical decision making.

a. _____

b. _____

c. _____

d. _____

e. _____

12. For the following scenarios, determine the type of ethical problem presented. Although these situations may present more than one ethical problem, choose only one possibility for each exercise.

A. Two sisters have arrived at a medical facility to discuss with the attending physician the course of action they should take regarding their dying father. Mr. Roberts, the patient, is no longer responsive. Cassandra wants to continue all possible medical treatment to keep her father alive. Janet insists that her father would not want his life prolonged by artificial means. Mr. Roberts did not give either sister a power of attorney, and he did not leave a written record of his wishes on this issue.

a. Type of ethical problem

_____

_____

b. What should you do if one of the sisters asks for your personal opinion on her father's situation? What do you do if you feel very differently from the daughter in this situation?

_____

_____

_____

B. Dr. Ho is the chief of staff at a regional medical center. His specialty is oncology, and the hospital is considering the construction of a cancer center as part of a multimillion-dollar project. One of Dr. Patrick's partners, Dr. Adams, is vehemently opposed to the project because of the cost to the local taxpayers who support the hospital. Dr. Adams has threatened to leave the practice unless Dr. Patrick votes against the project. Dr. Patrick wants the center to be built, but he also realizes that if Dr. Adams leaves, the practice will suffer a drastic loss of income.

a. Type of ethical problem

_____

_____

b. How would you handle an ethical decision that has an equal number of pros and cons?

_____

_____

_____

13. Summarize the opinions of the Council on Ethical and Judicial Affairs (CEJA) on the following ethical issues. Include in your description how these ethical opinions might affect an entry-level medical assistant.

a. Physicians and Allied Health Professions

_____

_____

_____

b. Preventing, Identifying, and Treating Violence and Abuse

_____

_____

_____

c. HIV Testing

_____

_____

_____

d. Organ Donation

_____

_____

_____

e. Confidentiality

_____

_____

_____

f. Fees and Charges

_____

_____

_____

g. Conflicts of Interest

_____

_____

_____

14. How should the medical assistant ethically manage a conflict of interest with his or her physician employer?

_____

_____

_____

15. Explain why confidentiality is critical in the medical environment.

_____

_____

_____

16. Explain the recommendations of the American College of Physicians regarding conflicts of interest.

_____

_____

_____

Read the case studies and answer the questions that follow.

1. Robert is a patient who has tested positive for the human immunodeficiency virus (HIV). Because he wants to protect all healthcare workers involved in his care, he informs you of his HIV status when he makes his first appointment. What should you do with this information? How will you interact with Robert when he comes to his first appointment?

   _____

   _____

   _____

2. You are employed by a cardiologist who has just returned from a cruise that was sponsored by a major pharmaceutical company. The physician frequently writes prescriptions for the company's cardiovascular drugs although many patients have told you they cannot afford the medication. How should you handle this potential conflict of interest? Ultimately, what can you do to advocate for patients in the practice?

   _____

   _____

   _____

3. You discover a co-worker taking drug samples out of the medication room. She tells you her son has an ear infection and she can't afford the antibiotics ordered for him. How should you manage this situation? What is the ethical response?

   _____

   _____

   _____

WORKPLACE APPLICATION

Stepping into the medical environment, where confidentiality is so important, may be a difficult adjustment for some new medical assistants. In any medical facility, you must think before speaking. At times, discussing patients and their conditions will not be appropriate. How can you change your way of thinking and be constantly aware of the constraints that patient confidentiality places on the discussion of patient information?

INTERNET ACTIVITIES

Choose one or more of these activities and share your results with the class, if appropriate.

1. Review the website for the Health Insurance Portability and Accountability Act (HIPAA) and download the quick fact sheets. Study this information to gain a basic knowledge of HIPAA guidelines and discuss with the class.

2. Discuss ethics in the classroom. How do medical assistant students perform ethically while completing their education? Research this issue on the Internet and talk about it in class.

3. Read the Code of Ethics from the AAMA in your textbook. Research codes of ethics for healthcare workers online. What are their similarities?

4. Research the requirements for reporting positive HIV tests in your state. Share your findings with the class.

Student Name _____ Date _____

AFFECTIVE COMPETENCY: XI.A1. RECOGNIZE THE IMPACT PERSONAL ETHICS AND MORALS MAY HAVE ON THE DELIVERY OF HEALTHCARE

Explanation: Student must achieve a minimum score of 3 in each category to achieve competency.

Both personal and professional ethics contribute to the way the medical assistant approaches a patient. However, the medical assistant must never force his or her personal beliefs and values on the patient or family members. Personal beliefs and professional ethics must be kept separate, allowing patients to make their own decisions about healthcare and enabling respectful patient care. Practicing ethical patient care is extremely important when working with a diverse patient population.

Empathy is the key to creating a caring, therapeutic environment. A medical assistant who is empathetic respects the individuality of the patient and attempts to see the person's health problem through his or her eyes, recognizing the effect of all holistic factors on the patient's well-being. Empathetic sensitivity to diversity first requires those interested in healthcare to examine their own values, beliefs, and actions; you cannot treat all patients with caring and respect until you first recognize and evaluate personal biases. We think and act a certain way for many reasons. The first step in understanding the process is to evaluate your individual value system.

Many different factors influence the development of a value system. Value systems begin as learned beliefs and behaviors. Families and cultural influences shape the way we respond to a diverse society. Other factors that influence reactions include socioeconomic and educational backgrounds. To develop therapeutic relationships, you must recognize your own value system to determine whether it could affect your method of interaction. Preconceived ideas about people because of their race, religion, income level, ethnic origin, sexual orientation, or gender can act as barriers to the development of a therapeutic relationship. You will be unable to treat your patients empathetically unless you can connect with them in some way. Personal biases or prejudices are monumental barriers to the development of therapeutic relationships and the delivery of ethical patient care.

Using the following case studies from the Medicine and Ethics chapter, role-play with your partner how you would examine the effect that personal ethics and morals may have on the delivery of healthcare.

You are responsible for recording an in-depth interview of a 21-year-old single mother who is pregnant with her third child. Demonstrate how you would ethically interact with this patient.

Karl Owenson is being seen today for a severe lung infection and requests that his partner, Tim, be present during the examination.

Sven Olstein is a sexually active 28-year-old who is being treated for his fourth episode of chlamydia.

Scoring Criteria (1 Thru 4)	Excellent Evidence of Learning 4	Adequate Evidence of Learning 3	Limited Evidence of Learning 2	Unacceptable Evidence of Learning 1	Score Attempt 1	Score Attempt 2	Score Attempt 3
Recognizes the effect that personal ethics and morals may have on the delivery of healthcare	Student demonstrates the highest level of examination of the effect that personal ethics and morals may have on the delivery of healthcare	Student demonstrates mastery level of examination of the effect that personal ethics and morals may have on the delivery of healthcare	Student is developing competency in examination of the effect that personal ethics and morals may have on the delivery of healthcare	Student demonstrates the main concepts of examination of the effect that personal ethics and morals may have on the delivery of healthcare but does not perform them adequately			

74

Scoring Criteria (1 Thru 4)	Excellent Evidence of Learning 4	Adequate Evidence of Learning 3	Limited Evidence of Learning 2	Unacceptable Evidence of Learning 1	Score Attempt 1	Score Attempt 2	Score Attempt 3
Provides professional and compassionate care to the patient regardless of personal ethics and morals	Student demonstrates the highest level of professional and compassionate care to the patient regardless of personal ethics and morals	Student demonstrates mastery level of professional and compassionate care to the patient regardless of personal ethics and morals	Student demonstrates limited professional and compassionate care to the patient because of personal ethics and morals	Student fails to demonstrate professional and compassionate care to the patient because of personal ethics and morals			

Instructor Comments:

PROCEDURE 7-1. DEVELOP A PLAN FOR SEPARATING PERSONAL AND PROFESSIONAL ETHICS: RECOGNIZE THE IMPACT PERSONAL ETHICS AND MORALS HAVE ON THE DELIVERY OF HEALTHCARE

MAERB/CAAHEP COMPETENCIES: XI.P.1.
ABHES COMPETENCIES: 4.g.

TASK: Determine one's ethical and moral views before having to confront an ethical decision.
Using the following case studies, role-play with your partner issues of personal and professional ethical behavior and how personal ethics and morals can affect the delivery of healthcare. Role-play each case as a separate ethical problem and apply the ethical decision-making process to each.

1. While you are gathering information from a new patient he informs you that he is HIV positive. Do you think this will affect your therapeutic relationship?
2. You are responsible for performing an in-depth diabetic education intervention with an individual with very poor hygiene. Will this cause a problem with your professional manner?
3. You are told by your office manager that an inmate of the county prison is scheduled for an appointment this afternoon. Do you think his status will affect your reaction to this patient?
4. You are attempting to gather insurance information from a 20-year-old patient who brought her two young children with her to the office today. She is a single mother who is pregnant with her third child and receives public assistance. What do you think? Will you have difficulty being empathetic?

EQUIPMENT AND SUPPLIES:
- Pen and paper
- Copy of the AAMA's Medical Assisting Code of Ethics

Standards: Complete the procedure and all critical steps in _____ minutes with a minimum score of 85% within three attempts.

Scoring: Divide the points earned by the total possible points. Failure to perform a critical step, indicated by an asterisk (*), results in an unsatisfactory overall score.

Time began _____ **Time ended** _____ **Total minutes:** _____

Steps	Possible Points	Attempt 1	Attempt 2	Attempt 3
1. Set aside time to study and consider the ethical issues outlined in this chapter.	5	_____	_____	_____
2. For each issue, make notes on your personal thoughts, paying particular attention to whether you agree with the AAMA's Medical Assisting Code of Ethics.	5	_____	_____	_____
3. Look at each issue as a separate ethical problem and apply the ethical decision-making process to each.	5	_____	_____	_____
4. Gather relevant information by researching each problem.	5	_____	_____	_____
5. Identify the type of ethical problem that each issue represents.	5	_____	_____	_____
*6. Determine your personal view on each issue to recognize how personal ethics and morals can affect the delivery of quality patient care.	10	_____	_____	_____
*7. Determine the ethical approach to use. Knowing the type of problem that each ethical issue represents helps the medical assistant determine the best approach to each decision.	10	_____	_____	_____

Steps	Possible Points	Attempt 1	Attempt 2	Attempt 3
8. Explore practical alternatives. Considering all practical alternatives helps the medical assistant make the best ethical decisions.	10	_____	_____	_____
9. Decide your personal stand on each issue.	5	_____	_____	_____
*10. Determine the position of the Medical Assisting Code of Ethics on each issue.	10	_____	_____	_____
11. Continue the process until each ethical issue has been addressed.	5	_____	_____	_____
*12. Refrain from placing personal ethical views on patients.	10	_____	_____	_____
*13. Interact with patients in a professional manner regardless of their or your own ethical views.	10	_____	_____	_____
14. Re-evaluate personal ethical views periodically and apply new knowledge and experience to determine whether ethical views have changed.	5	_____	_____	_____

Comments:

Points earned _____ ÷ 100 possible points = Score _____ % Score

Instructor's signature _____

PROCEDURE 7-2. RESPOND TO ISSUES OF CONFIDENTIALITY

CAAHEP COMPETENCIES: XI.P.2.
ABHES COMPETENCIES: 4.b., 4.f.

TASK: Ensure that medical assistants treat all information regarding patient care as completely confidential.

EQUIPMENT AND SUPPLIES:
- Patient's health record
- Copy of the Medical Assisting Code of Ethics
- Copy of the Medical Assisting Creed
- Copy of the Oath of Hippocrates (see the chapter, The Medical Assistant and the Healthcare Team)
- Copy of HIPAA guidelines (see the chapter, Medicine and Law)
- Notepad and pen

Select a student with whom to role-play as a patient. The patient should present with a situation in one of the case studies.

1. You work for a local OG/GYN and your best friend tells you her brother's wife is having an affair and your friend wants you to find out if she is pregnant. You saw the woman in the office today and know that her pregnancy test is positive. How would you manage this situation?
2. An attorney calls the office today and requests that you send copies of a patient's health records to her office ASAP for a liability case. The patient has not signed a release form but the attorney tells you she doesn't need one because this is a legal matter. What would you do?
3. The mother of a 19-year-old patient calls today and wants you to release her son's laboratory test results. The son lives with her and is covered by her medical insurance but the mother is not included in the patient's Notice of Privacy Practices (NPP) form. Does the mother have the right to this information?

Standards: Complete the procedure and all critical steps in _____ minutes with a minimum score of 85% within three attempts.

Scoring: Divide the points earned by the total possible points. Failure to perform a critical step, indicated by an asterisk (*), results in an unsatisfactory overall score.

Time began _____ **Time ended** _____ **Total minutes:** _____

Steps	Possible Points	Attempt 1	Attempt 2	Attempt 3
1. Read through each document, paying particular attention to the references to confidentiality.	5	_____	_____	_____
2. Select a student with whom to role-play as a patient. The patient should present with a situation or an illness he or she wants to keep confidential.	5	_____	_____	_____
*3. Identify each patient by name and date of birth.	10	_____	_____	_____
4. Take the patient to a private exam room or other area suitable for a private conversation and attend to his or her needs and questions.	5	_____	_____	_____
5. Listen carefully to what the patient says, taking notes if necessary, asking clarifying questions, and using restatement to clear up any misunderstandings.	5	_____	_____	_____

Steps	Possible Points	Attempt 1	Attempt 2	Attempt 3
6. Assure the patient that his or her concerns and health issues are confidential.	10	_____	_____	_____
7. Explain to the patient that information shared with you cannot be kept from the provider.	10	_____	_____	_____
*8. Discuss the information with the practitioner or ask the provider to speak personally with the patient, depending on which is appropriate to the circumstances.	15	_____	_____	_____
9. Instruct the patient according to the provider's orders, if necessary.	5	_____	_____	_____
*10. Document the patient's concerns, information given by the patient, and the provider's orders in the health record.	15	_____	_____	_____
*11. Do not share information about the patient with anyone not directly related to the patient's care.	15	_____	_____	_____

Comments:

Points earned _____ ÷ **100 possible points = Score** _____ **% Score**

Instructor's signature _____

8 Technology and Written Communication

Technology in the Medical Office

VOCABULARY REVIEW

Fill in the blanks with the correct vocabulary terms from this chapter.

1. Jane must do a system _____ _____ each evening to copy and archive computer data that could be used if a compromise occurs.

2. Dr. Jones uses the _____ _____ _____ to find information on a patient's visit to a specialist and to the emergency department at the local hospital.

3. Sally must install a new version of the _____, which will act as a filter between the network and the Internet.

4. Employees are not allowed onto social _____ sites during work hours, and the computers may not allow employees to access these Internet sites.

5. The receptionist uses a _____ _____ or privacy screen on his monitor to prevent unauthorized people from viewing information on the monitor.

6. Dr. Black uses her tablet that has _____ _____ _____ apps and tools when she is working with patients.

7. The office employees use _____ _____ _____ for scheduling, billing, and accounting tasks.

8. The providers use _____ to send prescriptions from the electronic health record (EHR) to pharmacies.

9. Computer hardware and software that perform data analysis, storage, and archiving are called a(n) _____ _____.

10. The computer process of changing encrypted text to readable or plain text after a user enters a secret key or password is called _____.

11. The system in the medical facility that links personal computers with peripheral devices to share information and resources is called a(n) _____ _____.

12. _____ _____ are used to monitor users' activity within software, including additions, deletions, and viewing of electronic records.

13. The communication system for connecting several computers together so that information can be shared is called a(n) _____.

14. The _____ _____ acts like the computer's software administrator, whereas the _____ _____ helps the computer to function and includes file managers and screensavers.

15. _____ software is used to protect computers against viruses.

SKILLS AND CONCEPTS

Part I: Matching Exercises

Match the following terms with their definitions.

1. _____ Approximately 1 billion bytes   a. Terabyte

2. _____ Approximately 1 trillion bytes   b. Kilobyte

3. _____ 1024 bytes   c. Megabyte

4. _____ Character (e.g., number, letter)   d. Byte

5. _____ Approximately 1 million bytes   e. Gigabyte

Part II: Input, Output, and Storage Devices

Label each of the following as an input, output, or storage device.

1. Mouse	Input	Output	Storage
2. Keyboard	Input	Output	Storage
3. Printer	Input	Output	Storage
4. Scanner	Input	Output	Storage
5. Jump drive	Input	Output	Storage
6. Touchpad	Input	Output	Storage
7. Blu-ray disk	Input	Output	Storage
8. Touch screen	Input	Output	Storage
9. Webcam	Input	Output	Storage
10. Signature pad	Input	Output	Storage
11. Monitor	Input	Output	Storage

Part III: Internal Parts of the Computer

Provide the name of the computer part described in the sentences that follow.

1. Responsible for interpreting and executing commands from the software; also called the "brains" of the computer

   _____

2. Platform where all the internal computer parts are attached

   _____

3. Memory used when the computer boots up

   _____

4. Contains instructions for opening programs; computer scans this memory first to see if data exist there before looking elsewhere

   _____

5. Working memory that is required for the computer to operate; holds data that are currently being used and empties when the power is turned off

   _____

6. Device that reads and writes on a hard disk

_____

7. More expensive, but faster and more reliable than an HDD

_____

8. Can read or read and save data on CDs, DVDs, and BDs

_____

9. Allows the audio information to be sent to headphones or speakers (provide all three names)

_____

10. Allows graphical information to be sent to the monitor or the projector (provide all three names)

_____

Part IV: Secondary Storage Devices

Describe the following terms related to storage devices.

1. Secondary storage devices

_____

_____

2. Magnetic storage devices

_____

_____

3. Optical storage devices

_____

_____

4. Flash storage devices

_____

_____

5. Cloud storage

_____

_____

Part V: Short Answer

1. Describe three ways to protect the computer and all peripheral devices from damage.

 a. _____

 b. _____

 c. _____

2. Describe what to do if liquids spill on the keyboard.

_____

_____

Chapter **8** **Technology and Written Communication**

3. Explain how to clean the casing of a printer or other hardware device.

_____

_____

4. Discuss how to clean a nonglare or antiglare screen on a monitor.

_____

_____

5. Describe why it is important to disinfect keyboards in a medical facility.

_____

_____

6. Discuss how to handle CDs, DVDs, and BDs.

_____

_____

7. For an ergonomically correct workstation, describe how the chair must fit the user.

_____

_____

_____

_____

8. Explain the position of the monitor in an ergonomically correct workstation.

_____

_____

9. Discuss the advantages of using an ergonomic keyboard.

_____

_____

10. Differentiate between system software and application software.

_____

_____

_____

_____

11. Differentiate between electronic medical records (EMRs) and practice management software.

_____

_____

_____

_____

12. Explain the importance of computer network security and data backup activities performed in the medical office.

_____

_____

_____

_____

13. Discuss advances in technology that affect the medical office.

_____

_____

_____

_____

14. Discuss applications of electronic technology in the medical office.

_____

_____

_____

_____

CASE STUDY

Read the case study and answer the questions that follow.

Brooke Comis works for Dr. Tomms as a clinical medical assistant. She is a former office computer specialist who worked in the computer field for 12 years before she entered medical assisting school. She changed career fields because she always wanted to work in healthcare and liked working with people. Unfortunately, she is the only person in the office who is knowledgeable about computers, the Internet, and networking. Whenever a computer is not functioning correctly or a problem occurs with the network, Dr. Tomms asks Brooke to fix it. When he decided to buy new computers, he expected Brooke to assemble all of them and set up a new network. Brooke gets more and more irate each time she is asked to perform these duties because she is not compensated other than her normal hourly pay. She knows that if Dr. Tomms paid someone to do this work, it would cost him more than her monthly salary. Brooke is not certain how to handle this situation. What should she do first? How should she approach the physician? Should she refuse to perform computer work? What could happen if she refuses?

_____

_____

_____

_____

_____

_____

_____

_____

Complete one or more of these activities and, if appropriate, share your results with the class.

1. Assume that you have been selected to order a new computer system for the healthcare facility. The clinic's personnel include three providers, six administrative personnel, and four clinical assistants, plus you, the office manager. Describe the minimal equipment needed. Consider printers, Internet access, scanners, and wireless needs. Investigate computers using the Internet and prepare a folder with photos or specifications that detail the equipment you have selected.

2. Completely disconnect a computer, including all cords and peripheral devices. Make sure to label the cords on each end as to where they should be placed, before disconnecting all cords. Reconnect the cords to the computer and peripheral devices. Turn the computer on and use each device to make certain that it has been connected the right way. Students may want to complete this activity on a home computer, or the instructor may set up a computer in the classroom to disconnect and reconnect. Students should write a paragraph describing their experiences with this project.

INTERNET ACTIVITY OPTIONS

Complete one or more of these activities and, if appropriate, share your results with the class.

1. Use the Internet to locate a company that sells computers in your geographic area. Explore the site. Find a computer that you might consider purchasing, then answer the following questions.

   a. How much RAM and ROM does the system have? _____

   b. What software, if any, comes with the system? _____

   c. What is the total cost before taxes are applied? _____

2. Search the Internet using the key words "evaluating Internet health information tutorial" and view the tutorial. Describe five items you can evaluate when looking at online health websites.

3. You are working in a dermatology office with two providers and three other medical assistants. The department moved to a practice management system and an EHR last year. Currently, each provider and medical assistant has his or her own laptop, but the group has decided to investigate other computer devices that might be able to replace the laptops. Investigate portable computer devices using the Internet and prepare a folder with photos or specifications that detail the equipment you have selected.

Written Communication in the Medical Office

VOCABULARY REVIEW

Fill in the blanks with the correct vocabulary terms from this chapter.

1. A(n) _____ is a word or phrase for a person, place, thing, or idea.

2. A(n) _____ is a word or a phrase that shows action or a state of being.

3. A(n) _____ is a phrase without a main clause.

4. A(n) _____ is a word or group of words that describes a noun or pronoun.

5. _____ are words that sound alike.

6. The _____ _____ is usually located in the header of a letter and provides the clinic's name and address and may include other contact information.

7. The _____ _____ is the part of the letter that contains the recipient's name, title, department, agency, and address.

8. The _____ is the greeting in a letter.

9. Bob is printing a letter and knows that _____ _____ is the most common layout for letters because the height of the paper is longer than the width.

10. Keith must use _____ software to compress files he is e-mailing.

SKILLS AND CONCEPTS

Part I: Identify the Errors

Identify the error(s), then rewrite the sentence on the line correcting the error.

1. To patients arrived at the same time.

   _____

2. Zac the receptionist greet the patients when they arrived.

   _____

3. My appointment is on August 17th 20XX.

   _____

4. Yesterday, Betsy and Sue work with Dr Jones.

   _____

5. Marie and me arrived early at the medical office.

   _____

6. Yes i will need your new insurance card.

   _____

7. Thank you katie for all your hard work.

   _____

8. The mother father and son arrived late for there appointments.

   _____

9. Wear did the patient go.

   _____

10. There parents are talking with the provider.

    _____

Part II: Short Answers

1. Describe the paper, margins, and line spacing used in professional letters.

   _____

   _____

   _____

   _____

2. What is the purpose of the reference line in a professional letter?

_____

_____

3. How would you compose a greeting for a professional letter to John White?

_____

4. What are two ways a reference notation would be typed if Sally James were typing a letter for Dr. Mike Vast?

_____

5. Describe why "c." would be used as a copy notation instead of "cc." to indicate a copy of the letter was sent to another person.

_____

_____

6. Name three items that should be on a continuation page.

a. _____

b. _____

c. _____

7. Describe the difference between "closed" and "open" punctuation in a letter.

_____

_____

8. Describe a full block letter format.

_____

_____

9. Describe the similarities and differences between the modified block letter format and the semi-block letter format.

_____

_____

_____

_____

10. List the four headings used in memorandums and include the correct punctuation.

a. _____

b. _____

c. _____

d. _____

Part III: Create Professional Letters

Using Procedure 8-1 as a guide, create letters for the following scenarios. Create your own letterhead in the header of the document. You are working at Walden-Martin Family Medical Clinic. The practice's address is 1234 Anystreet, Anytown, AL 12345. The phone number is 123-123-1234, and the fax number is 123-123-5678.

1. Use the full block letter format and create the following letter:

   Jean Burke, NP, has requested that you compose a letter to Janine Butler (DOB 04/25/1968) and let her know that her mammogram from last Wednesday was negative. She should make a follow-up appointment in 6 months. If she has any questions, she should call the office. Janine's address is: 37 Park West Avenue, Anytown, AL 12345-1234.

2. Use the full block letter format and create the following letter:

   James A. Martin, MD, has requested that you compose a letter to Celia Tapia (DOB 05/18/1970) and let her know that her Pap test from last Thursday was negative. She should make a follow-up appointment in 1 year. If she has any questions, she should call the office. Celia's address is: 12 Highland Court, Apt 101, Anytown, AL 12345-1234.

3. Use the modified block letter format with the center point variation and create the following letter:

   Julie Walden, MD, has requested that you compose a letter to the mother (Patricia Jackson) of Aaron Jackson (DOB 10/17/2011) and let her know that Aaron's left wrist radiograph was negative. He should continue wearing the wrist splint for the next 2 weeks. If he is not getting better or if she has questions, she should call the office. Patricia's address is: 555 McArthur Avenue, Anytown, AL 12345-1234.

4. Use the semi-block letter format with the right justified variation and create the following letter:

   Jean Burke, NP, has requested that you compose a letter to Ken Thomas (DOB 10/25/1961) and let him know that his urine culture is negative for growth. He should make a follow-up appointment for 2 weeks from his initial appointment. If he has any questions, he should call the office. Ken's address is 398 Larkin Avenue, Anytown, AL 12345-1234.

Part IV: Professional E-mail

Using Procedure 8-2 as a guide, create e-mails for the following scenarios. Your instructor will provide you with the e-mail address for your e-mails. You are a medical assistant working at Walden-Martin Family Medical Clinic. The practice's address is 1234 Anystreet, Anytown, AL 12345. The phone number is 123-123-1234, and the fax number is 123-123-5678. The clinic's name and contact information should be after your name in the closing section of the e-mail.

1. Create and send an e-mail appointment reminder:

   Johnny Parker (06/15/2010) has an appointment at 10:00 AM next Tuesday. Send his mother, Lisa Parker, an appointment reminder via e-mail. Johnny will be seeing Jean Burke, NP. The mother should bring in any medications that Johnny is currently taking.

2. Create and send an e-mail appointment reminder:

   Erma Willis (12/09/1947) has an appointment at 9:00 AM next Thursday. Send her an appointment reminder via e-mail. Erma will be seeing Julie Walden, MD. She should bring in any medications that she is currently taking.

3. Create and send an e-mail regarding a medication refill:

   Walter Biller (01/04/1970) had e-mailed requesting a refill on his atorvastatin, and he wanted to pick up the medication at Anytown Drug Store. Julie Walden, MD, asked you to contact Walter and let him know she sent the refill order to Anytown Drug Store. You should let him know that he should take 10 mg (1 tablet) every day. He will get a 90-day supply with three refills.

4. Create and send an e-mail regarding a medication refill:

   Norma Washington (08/01/1944) had e-mailed requesting a refill on her atenolol, and she wanted to pick up the medication at Anytown Drug Store. James Martin, MD, asked you to contact Norma and let her know he sent the refill order to Anytown Drug Store. You should let her know that she should take 25 mg (1 tablet) every day. She will get a 60-day supply with five refills.

Read the case study and answer the questions that follow.

Barbara recently graduated as a medical assistant and obtained employment at a local provider's office. She and the office manager have been at odds since Barbara redesigned several forms that had been in use at the clinic but had been copied over and over again and looked quite unprofessional. Barbara did not ask permission to redo the forms; she was attempting to help and to make a good impression. Since that incident, the office manager has given Barbara two written reprimands for minor issues.

1. What should Barbara do?

_____

_____

_____

2. How could she have prevented this situation from the beginning?

_____

_____

_____

3. Is the office manager at fault?

_____

_____

_____

WORKPLACE APPLICATION OPTION

Complete this activity and, if appropriate, share your results with the class.

Collect several documents from various healthcare facilities. Compare the quality of the documents. Do they make a good first impression? Are they clearly copies that have been made over and over again? Grade the documents and revise those that are graded below a B so that they present a positive, professional image of the facility.

INTERNET ACTIVITY OPTIONS

Complete one or more of these activities and, if appropriate, share your results with the class.

1. Research professional e-mail etiquette. Describe five ways you can improve your written communication with patients and professionals.

2. Research confidentiality and e-mails with patients. Describe how to keep the e-mails to patients within the guidelines of HIPAA.

3. Research the two-letter postal abbreviations for the states. Write each address provided as it should appear on an envelope. Use only approved U.S. Postal Service standard street abbreviations and the two-letter postal abbreviation for states.

   a. Walden-Martin Family Medical Clinic, 1234 Any Street, Anytown, Alabama 14453

   _____

   _____

   _____

b. John Smith, 383 E. Center, Anytown, Nebraska 13333-2232

_____

_____

_____

c. Sally Black, 39291 S. Parkway, Anytown, Wisconsin 54334-6443

_____

_____

_____

d. Jeff Jones, 454 Boulevard, Anytown, Minnesota 49932-1234

_____

_____

_____

e. Sam House, 599 State Highway, Anytown, Illinois 69532-1651

_____

_____

_____

4. Use the zip code look-up tool on www.usps.com to find the zip codes for the following cities. Write the zip code on the line to the right of the city.

a. Best, TX   _____

b. Beauty, KY   _____

c. Celebration, FL   _____

d. Hot Coffee, MS   _____

e. Success, MO   _____

f. Carefree, AZ   _____

g. Pie Town, NM   _____

h. Embarrass, WI   _____

i. Sandwich, MA   _____

j. Oddville, KY   _____

k. Peculiar, MO   _____

l. Ham Lake, MN   _____

m. Tea, SD   _____

Chapter **8** **Technology and Written Communication**

5. Use the zip code look-up tool on www.usps.com to find the zip codes with the four-digit extension for the following addresses. Write your answer on the line to the right of the address.

   a. State Capitol   _____

      600 Dexter Ave

      Montgomery AL

   b. Capitol Building   _____

      600 E Boulevard Ave

      Bismarck ND

   c. State Capitol   _____

      210 Capitol Ave

      Hartford CT

   d. State of Florida   _____

      400 S Monroe St

      Tallahassee FL

   e. 2300 N Lincoln Blvd Rm 212   _____

      Oklahoma City OK

Name _____ Date _____ Score _____

PROCEDURE 8-1. COMPOSE PROFESSIONAL CORRESPONDENCE USING ELECTRONIC TECHNOLOGY: COMPOSE A PROFESSIONAL BUSINESS LETTER

MAERB/CAAHEP COMPETENCIES: V.P.8.
ABHES COMPETENCIES: 7.a., 7.b.

TASK: Compose a professional letter using technology

EQUIPMENT AND SUPPLIES:
- Computer with word processing software and printer
- Paper or letterhead paper
- #10 Envelope
- Patient's health record

Standards: Complete the procedure and all critical steps in _____ minutes with a minimum score of 85% within three attempts.

Scoring: Divide the points earned by the total possible points. Failure to perform a critical step, indicated by an asterisk (*), results in an unsatisfactory overall score.

Time began _____ Time ended _____ Total minutes: _____

Steps	Possible Points	Attempt 1	Attempt 2	Attempt 3
1. Obtain the intended recipient's contact information and determine the message to convey to the recipient.	5	_____	_____	_____
2. Using the computer and word processing software, compose the letter using one of the three business letter formats. If using blank paper, create a letterhead in the header of the document and include the clinic's name, street address or Post Office box, city, state, and zip code.	10	_____	_____	_____
3. Type the date in the correct location using the correct format. Have one blank line between the date line and the last line of the letterhead.	5	_____	_____	_____
4. Type the inside address using the correct spelling, punctuation, and location for the information. Leave one to nine blank lines between the date and the inside address, depending on the location of the body of the letter.	10	_____	_____	_____
5. Starting on the second line below the inside address, type the salutation using the correct format.	5	_____	_____	_____
6. Type the message in the body of the letter using the proper location and format. There should be a blank line after the salutation and between each paragraph. The message should be clear, concise, and professional. Use proper grammar, punctuation, capitalization, and sentence structure.	10	_____	_____	_____

Steps	Possible Points	Attempt 1	Attempt 2	Attempt 3
7. Type a proper closing, leaving one blank line between the last line of the body and the closing. Use the correct format and location.	5	_____	_____	_____
8. Type the signature block using the correct format and location. If the typist is preparing the letter for a physician, the typist will also need to include a reference notation. There should be four blank lines between the closing and the signature block.	10	_____	_____	_____
*9. Spell-check and proofread the document. Check for proper tone, grammar, punctuation, capitalization, and sentence structure. Check for proper spacing between the parts of the letter.	10	_____	_____	_____
10. Make any final corrections. Print the document on letterhead or on regular paper on which you inserted the letterhead.	5	_____	_____	_____
11. Address the envelope either using the computer and word processing software or with a pen following the correct format. After addressing the envelope, give the letter with the envelope attached to the provider to review and sign.	10	_____	_____	_____
12. File a copy of the letter in the paper medical record or upload an electronic copy of the letter to the EHR.	10	_____	_____	_____
13. Fold the letter using the correct technique and place in the envelope.	5	_____	_____	_____

Comments:

Points earned _____ ÷ 100 possible points = **Score** _____ **% Score**

Instructor's signature _____

PROCEDURE 8-2. COMPOSE PROFESSIONAL CORRESPONDENCE UTILIZING ELECTRONIC TECHNOLOGY: COMPOSE A PROFESSIONAL E-MAIL

MAERB/CAAHEP COMPETENCIES: V.P.8.
ABHES COMPETENCIES: 7.a., 7.b.

TASK: Compose a professional e-mail that conveys the message clearly, concisely, and accurately to the reader.

EQUIPMENT AND SUPPLIES:
- Computer with e-mail software
- Patient's health record

Standards: Complete the procedure and all critical steps in _____ minutes with a minimum score of 85% within three attempts.

Scoring: Divide the points earned by the total possible points. Failure to perform a critical step, indicated by an asterisk (*), results in an unsatisfactory overall score.

Time began _____ **Time ended** _____ **Total minutes:** _____

Steps	Possible Points	Attempt 1	Attempt 2	Attempt 3
1. Obtain the intended recipient's contact information and determine the message to convey to the recipient.	5	_____	_____	_____
2. Using the computer and e-mail software, key in the recipient's e-mail address. If the e-mail has two recipients, separate the first name using a semicolon (;). Double-check the e-mail addresses for accuracy.	5	_____	_____	_____
3. Type in a subject, keeping it simple but focused on the contents of the e-mail.	10	_____	_____	_____
4. Type a formal greeting using correct punctuation.	10	_____	_____	_____
5. Type the message in the body of the e-mail using proper grammar, punctuation, capitalization, and sentence structure. Avoid abbreviations. The message should be clear, concise, and professional.	20	_____	_____	_____
6. Finish the e-mail with closing remarks.	10	_____	_____	_____
7. Type a closing followed by your name and title on the next line. Include the clinic's name and contact information below your name.	10	_____	_____	_____
*8. Spell-check and proofread the e-mail. Check for proper tone, grammar, punctuation, capitalization, and sentence structure. Check for proper spacing between the parts of the e-mail.	20	_____	_____	_____
9. Make any final revisions, select any features to apply to the e-mail, and then send the e-mail.	5	_____	_____	_____
10. Print a copy of the e-mail to be filed in the paper medical record or upload an electronic copy of the e-mail to the EHR.	5	_____	_____	_____

Comments:

Points earned _____ ÷ **100 possible points = Score** _____ **% Score**

Instructor's signature _____

9 | Telephone Techniques

VOCABULARY REVIEW

1. The office manager cautions the medical assistants to avoid _____, because most patients do not understand complicated medical terms.

2. The highness or lowness of sound is called its _____.

3. When speaking on the phone or in public, Dr. Conn knows that he should avoid _____ speech to keep the listeners interested and enthusiastic about what he has to say.

4. The utterance of articulate clear sounds is _____.

5. Dr. Beard ordered the laboratory tests _____ so that the results would be reported to him immediately.

6. Mackenzie has learned to be _____ when she speaks with patients on the phone so that she maintains a good relationship with them.

7. Dr. Lightfoot prefers that the receptionist _____ all his calls so that he can concentrate on the patients in the office during their examinations.

8. Patients have expressed that they would like to be able to talk to a real person when calling the office after hours. The office manager is considering using a(n) _____ to address patient concerns.

9. When the receptionist is not sure if the patient should be seen that day they would transfer the call to the _____ area.

10. _____ _____ _____ provides callers with a menu of choices to be directed to the correct department.

SKILLS AND CONCEPTS

Part I: Answering Incoming Calls and Taking Phone Messages

For each of the following scenarios, three questions to ask the patient, determine who should receive the message, and what actions need to be taken for proper follow-through. Clinical questions may be included but are not required.
   Staff Members at Dr. Julie Beard's Office:

Physician	Dr. Julie Beard
Office Manager	Julia Carpenter
Clinical Medical Assistant	Trina Martinez
Clinical Medical Assistant	Dean Howell
Scheduling Assistant	Stephanie Dickson
Receptionist	Ginny Holloway
Insurance Biller and Medical Records	Gloria Richardson

1. Message retrieved from the answering machine, "Hello, this is Peter Young. I saw Dr. Beard on Monday about a rash on my forearms. This thing isn't getting any better, and the cream she prescribed for me isn't helping the itching, and it's very uncomfortable. Is there anything else we can do to help it? My number is 972-555-9873." The message was received at 7:30 am on Thursday, February 3.

   - Who should receive this message?

     _____

   - Questions to ask the patient when returning the call:

     _____

     _____

     _____

   - What action should be taken after speaking with the patient?

     _____

     _____

     _____

     _____

     _____

     _____

     _____

2. Gerald Morris calls Dr. Beard's office today to ask whether his insurance has paid for his last office visit. He is an established patient and has worked as a city police officer for more than 10 years. After asking to place Mr. Morris on hold, you pull up his account on the computer. No insurance payment has been credited to his account, and a note indicates that his insurance was not in effect at the time of his office visit. Mr. Morris asks you to check with the insurance company and call him back, because he is concerned about resolving this issue. His phone number is 972-555-8824. This call was received at 3:45 pm on September 4.

   - Who should receive this message?

     _____

   - Questions to ask the patient:

     _____

     _____

     _____

   - What action should be taken after speaking with the patient?

     _____

     _____

     _____

     _____

3. Mr. Juan Ross calls to get his prescription for Ambien refilled. His pharmacy is Wolfe Drug, and the drugstore phone number is 214-555-4523. Mr. Ross is allergic to penicillin. His phone number is 214-555-2377. Mr. Ross's message was received on July 23 at 10:15 am.

- Who should receive this message?

  _____

- Questions to ask the patient:

  _____

  _____

  _____

  _____

- What action should be taken after speaking with the patient?

  _____

  _____

  _____

  _____

4. Message retrieved from the answering machine, "This is Sarah at Cline Meador Lab with a STAT laboratory report. It is 9:35 am on November 16. The patient's name is Laura Williamson, date of birth January 14, 1984 and her WBC count is 18,000. Please notify Dr. Beard immediately. The laboratory phone number is 800-555-3333 and my extension is 255. If she has any questions, please have her give me a call. Thanks."

- Who should receive this message?

  _____

- Questions to ask Sarah:

  _____

  _____

  _____

  _____

  _____

- What action should be taken after speaking with Sarah?

  _____

  _____

  _____

  _____

5. Judy Jordan has migraine headaches and occasionally takes hydrocodone to relieve the pain. Dr. Beard leaves the office for the weekend at noon on Friday, and office policy dictates that she is not to be paged except in emergencies. Patients with routine or lesser health issues are to be instructed to make an appointment to come in and see the physician or to go to the emergency department. Ms. Jordan calls at 4:45 pm on Friday afternoon, March 9, after Dr. Beard has left the office. She requests that the staff authorize a refill for her pain medicine and insists on speaking to the office manager, who currently is in a meeting. Ms. Jordan's phone number is 214-555-9822.

- Who should receive this message?

  _____

- Questions to ask the patient when returning the call:

  _____

  _____

  _____

  _____

- What action should be taken after speaking with the patient?

  _____

  _____

  _____

6. Message retrieved from the answering machine, "Hello. My name is Christina Cawtel, and I was referred to your office by Dr. Preston for evaluation of an ovarian cyst. Today is Wednesday, October 4, and it is 8 am. I would like to make an appointment for early next week if possible. My phone number is 817-555-9325. Oh, and by the way, I need to know if you are a provider for Aetna, because my company just changed to their managed care plan. I probably need to have a mammogram, too, and want to see whether you will order it before I come in for the appointment. Thanks."

- Who should receive this message?

  _____

- Questions to ask Ms. Cawtel when returning the call:

  _____

  _____

  _____

  _____

- What action should be taken after speaking with the patient?

  _____

  _____

  _____

7. "My name is Janeen Shaw, and I am Dr. Beard's patient. It is just before 2 pm and I am trying to reach you as soon as you open your office after lunch. I am having a hard time breathing, and I have stomach pains. I am hurting all over my upper body, on my chest, my arms, my neck, just everywhere. I'm sweating, and I'm very nauseated. I'm 45 years old, and I'm almost never ill. I wanted to find out if I can come in for an appointment today. Please call me back as soon as possible. My phone number is 601-555-3423. Thank you. Please call as soon as you can. I really feel awful."

- Who should receive this message?

  _____

- Questions to ask the patient when returning the call:

  _____

  _____

  _____

- What action should be taken after speaking with the patient?

  _____

  _____

  _____

Part II: Handling Difficult Calls

Indicate how you would handle the following difficult telephone calls.

1. Angry callers

   _____

   _____

   _____

   _____

2. Sales calls

   _____

   _____

   _____

3. Emergency calls

   _____

   _____

   _____

4. Unauthorized inquiry calls

   _____

   _____

   _____

Chapter **9** Telephone Techniques

5. Callers with complaints

_____

_____

_____

6. Callers who speak foreign languages or have heavy accents.

_____

_____

_____

_____

Part III: Answering the Telephone

Write an original phone greeting for each of these medical specialty offices.

1. Ophthalmologist

_____

_____

_____

2. Oncologist

_____

_____

_____

3. General practitioner

_____

_____

_____

4. Chiropractor

_____

_____

_____

5. Cosmetic surgeon

_____

_____

_____

6. Dermatologist

_____

_____

_____

Part IV: Fill-in-the-blank

1. Selecting which calls will be forwarded to the physician immediately is a process called _____.

2. The medical assistant should not eat, drink, or _____ while answering the office telephone.

3. The medical assistant must maintain patient _____ at all times, even when on the telephone.

5. Telephone calls should be answered by the _____ ring.

6. Unsatisfactory progress reports from patients should be directed to the _____.

7. _____ _____ help with communication when the healthcare facility has various locations.

Part V: Time Zones

1. When it is 3 pm in Dallas, it is _____ in Los Angeles, California.

2. When it is 2 pm in Washington state, it is _____ in New York City.

3. When it is 5 pm in Las Cruces, New Mexico, it is _____ in Flint, Michigan.

4. When it is 4 pm in Augusta, Maine, it is _____ in Columbia, South Carolina.

5. When it is 11 am in Biloxi, Mississippi, it is _____ in Chicago, Illinois.

Part VI: Telephone Technique

1. List five questions that might be asked of a patient who calls with an emergency situation:

_____

_____

_____

_____

_____

2. The phrase that often calms an angry patient is:

_____

3. Explain the procedure for transferring a phone call.

_____

_____

_____

_____

4. What should the medical assistant do if a caller refuses to identify himself or herself?

_____

_____

_____

5. List the seven components of a proper telephone message.

_____

_____

_____

_____

_____

_____

_____

CASE STUDY

1. Denise has been the receptionist for a moderately large clinic for the past 3 months. She replaced Dorothy, who retired. Denise has been overwhelmed with the calls to the clinic, and the office manager has spoken to her twice about missing calls. Denise insists that she is constantly on the phone answering and transferring calls. She is beginning to lose faith in herself, but as she considers why she is failing at her job, she realizes that two new physicians have joined the practice since Dorothy left, and numerous calls come to the clinic for those two physicians. Denise wants to suggest to the office manager that perhaps the time has come for a second receptionist, but she is unsure how to broach the subject. How can Denise begin her conversation with the office manager? What should she not do or say?

_____

_____

_____

_____

_____

WORKPLACE APPLICATION OPTIONS

1. Contact a clinic office manager and determine if he or she would allow you to shadow the office receptionist for a day. Take note of the types of calls that come into the clinic and how they are handled. Discuss the results of the visit with the class.

_____

_____

_____

2. Invite a receptionist to the class to discuss telephone techniques for the medical office.

_____

_____

_____

_____

3. Talk about appropriate voice mails that might be left when calling patients and/or business associates. Discuss how much the caller should say on a voice mail, and discuss what should be included in the message.

_____

_____

_____

_____

4. Talk about how calls from deaf patients, or other patients with disabilities, might be handled.

_____

_____

_____

_____

INTERNET ACTIVITIES

Use an online telephone directory to find the following telephone numbers for your city or community.

1. Nonemergency number for the police department

_____

2. Local social security office

_____

3. American Red Cross office

_____

4. Acute care hospital

_____

5. Meals on Wheels

_____

6. American Cancer Society

_____

7. Local senior center

_____

8. Local food bank

_____

9. Poison control

_____

10. Local child protective services

_____

PROCEDURE 9-1. DEMONSTRATE PROFESSIONAL TELEPHONE TECHNIQUES

MAERB/CAAHEP COMPETENCIES: V.P.6., V.P.7.
ABHES COMPETENCIES: 8.f.

TASK: To answer the telephone in a provider's office in a professional manner and respond to a request for action.

CASE STUDY: Charles Johnson, DOB 3/3/1958, an established patient of Dr. Martin has called to schedule an appointment to have his blood pressure checked. This will be a follow-up appointment that is 15 minutes in length. He is requesting that the appointment be on a Friday during his lunchtime between 11:00 and 12:00.

EQUIPMENT AND SUPPLIES:
- Telephone
- Pen or pencil
- Appointment book
- Computer
- Notepad

Standards: Complete the procedure and all critical steps in _____ minutes with a minimum score of 85% within three attempts.

Scoring: Divide the points earned by the total possible points. Failure to perform a critical step, indicated by an asterisk (*), results in an unsatisfactory overall score.

Time began _____ **Time ended** _____ **Total minutes:** _____

Steps	Possible Points	Attempt 1	Attempt 2	Attempt 3
1. Demonstrate telephone techniques by answering the telephone by the third ring.	10	_____	_____	_____
2. Speak distinctly with a pleasant tone and expression, at a moderate rate, and with sufficient volume for the person to understand every word.	10	_____	_____	_____
3. Identify the office and/or provider and yourself.	10	_____	_____	_____
*4. Verify the identity of the caller, and if using an electronic health record, bring the patient's medical record to the active screen of the computer.	20	_____	_____	_____
5. Screen the call if necessary.	10	_____	_____	_____
6. Apply active listening skills to assess whether the caller is distressed or agitated and to determine the concern to be addressed.	10	_____	_____	_____
7. Determine the needs of the caller and provide the requested information or service if possible. Provide the caller with excellent customer service. Be as helpful as possible. View the appointment schedule and determine the first Friday that would have an open appointment between 11:00 and 12:00.	10	_____	_____	_____

Steps	Possible Points	Attempt 1	Attempt 2	Attempt 3
8. Obtain sufficient patient information to schedule the appointment; full name, DOB, and insurance information. Repeat the date and time of the appointment to ensure that the patient has the correct information.	10	_____	_____	_____
9. Terminate the call in a pleasant manner and replace the receiver gently. Always allow the caller to hang up first.	10	_____	_____	_____

Comments:

Points earned _____ ÷ 100 possible points = **Score** _____ % **Score**

Instructor's signature _____

Name _____ Date _____ Score _____

PROCEDURE 9-2. DOCUMENT TELEPHONE MESSAGES AND REPORT RELEVANT INFORMATION CONCISELY AND ACCURATELY

MAERB/CAAHEP COMPETENCIES: V.P.6., V.P.7., V.P.11.
ABHES COMPETENCIES: 8.f.

TASK: To take an accurate telephone message and follow up on the requests made by the caller.

CASE STUDY: Norma Washington, DOB 8/1/1944, an established patient of Dr. Martin has called to report her blood pressure readings that she has been taking at home. Dr. Martin had made a recent change in her medication and wanted her to monitor her BP at home for 3 days and call in with the results. She has taken her blood pressure in the morning and in the evening for the past three days with the following results:

Day 1: 144/92 in the am, 156/94 in the pm.
Day 2: 136/84 in the am, 142/86 in the pm.
Day 3: 132/80 in the am, 138/82 in the pm.

EQUIPMENT AND SUPPLIES:
- Telephone
- Computer
- Message pad
- Pen or pencil
- Notepad

Standards: Complete the procedure and all critical steps in _____ minutes with a minimum score of 85% within three attempts.

Scoring: Divide the points earned by the total possible points. Failure to perform a critical step, indicated by an asterisk (*), results in an unsatisfactory overall score.

Time began _____ Time ended _____ Total minutes: _____

Steps	Possible Points	Attempt 1	Attempt 2	Attempt 3
1. Demonstrate telephone techniques by answering the telephone using the guidelines in Procedure 9-1.	10	_____	_____	_____
*2. Using a message pad or the computer, take the phone message (either on paper or by data entry into the computer) and obtain the following information:	20	_____	_____	_____
• Name of the person to whom the call is directed				
• Name of the person calling				
• Caller's telephone number				
• Reason for the call				
• Action to be taken				
• Date and time of the call				
• Initials of the person taking the call				
3. Apply active listening skills and repeat the information back to the caller after recording the message.	10	_____	_____	_____

109

Steps	Possible Points	Attempt 1	Attempt 2	Attempt 3
4. End the call and wait for the caller to hang up first.	10	_____	_____	_____
5. Document the telephone call with all pertinent information in the patient's health record.	10	_____	_____	_____
6. Deliver the phone message to the appropriate person.	10	_____	_____	_____
7. Follow up on important messages.	10	_____	_____	_____
8. If using paper messaging, keep old message books for future reference. Carbonless copies allow the facility to keep a permanent record of phone messages.	10	_____	_____	_____
9. File pertinent phone messages in the patient's health record. Make sure the computer record is closed after the documentation has been done.	10	_____	_____	_____

Comments:

Points earned _____ **+ 100 possible points = Score** _____ **% Score**

      Instructor's signature _____

10 Scheduling Appointments and Patient Processing

VOCABULARY REVIEW

1. Angela arranged for a short time _____ between Dr. Patrick's speaking engagement and his first afternoon appointment so that he would have time for lunch.

2. Gayle gained _____ in computers by taking Saturday classes on the newest software.

3. Olivia realized that she needed to take a(n) _____ medical terminology course before she could register for anatomy and physiology.

4. A patient who does not come to his or her scheduled appointment is considered a(n) _____ and must have this documented in the health record and in the appointment book.

5. Before using an appointment book, establish the _____ by marking all times that the provider is unavailable so that patients will not be scheduled during those times.

6. A patient from a neighboring clinic caused a(n) _____ in the hallway as he left because he disagreed with a billing statement.

7. _____ _____ are those who have been seen as patients in the clinic more than once.

8. The _____ among the staff at Dr. Wykowski's office has become strained since the office manager was terminated.

9. Cooperation and willingness to help other staff members are a(n) _____ part of the success of a practice.

10. Dr. Raleigh installed a(n) _____ system so that he could speak to the medical assistants in the front and back offices from the examination rooms.

11. Medical assistants must be aware of the _____ patients have of the office staff and take steps to ensure that it is a positive one.

12. Susan filed the laboratory reports in _____ order.

13. _____ information includes the patient's address, insurance information, and e-mail address.

14. Any _____ offered to a patient should be within the provider's orders, so make sure that a beverage with sugar is not offered to a diabetic.

15. Employees prefer to work in an office with a(n) _____ environment.

16. Dr. Lawson has a(n) _____ desire to serve her patients and promote wellness.

17. A secondary use of health information that cannot be reasonably prevented is called a(n) _____ _____.

18. Medical assistants may find it helpful to write a patient's name using _____ spelling to remember its pronunciation.

Part I: Appointment Reminder Cards

Practice completing appointment reminder cards on the forms provided. Students should be able to fill out the appointment cards with the information provided without difficulty.

1. Tai Yan has an appointment for August 23, 20XX, at 3:00 PM with Dr. Martin.

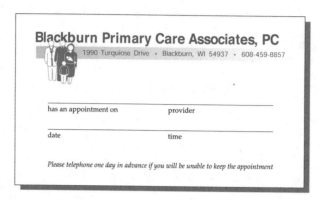

2. Diego Lupez has an appointment for May 1, 20XX, at 9:00 AM with Dr. Walden.

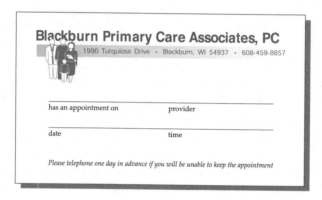

3. Julia Berkley has an appointment for June 13, 20XX, at 11:45 AM with Dr. Walden.

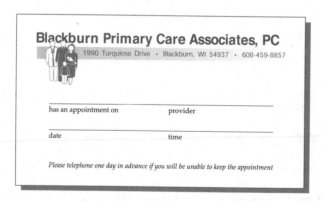

4. Monique Jones has an appointment for September 12, 20XX, at 2:40 PM with Jean Burke, NP.

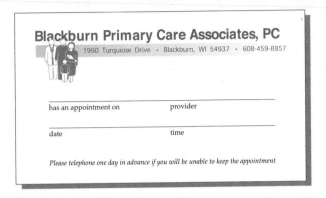

Blackburn Primary Care Associates, PC
1990 Turquiose Drive · Blackburn, WI 54937 · 608-459-8857

has an appointment on   provider

date   time

Please telephone one day in advance if you will be unable to keep the appointment

5. Ken Thomas has an appointment for December 15, 20XX, at 4:30 PM with Dr. Martin.

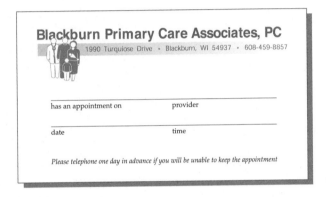

Blackburn Primary Care Associates, PC
1990 Turquiose Drive · Blackburn, WI 54937 · 608-459-8857

has an appointment on   provider

date   time

Please telephone one day in advance if you will be unable to keep the appointment

Part II: Guides for Scheduling

1. What three items must be considered when scheduling appointments?

_____

_____

_____

2. How can the medical assistant handle a provider who habitually spends more than the allotted time with patients?

_____

_____

_____

3. List one advantage and one disadvantage of using an appointment book for scheduling.

_____

_____

_____

4. List one advantage and one disadvantage of using a computer for scheduling.

_____

_____

_____

5. What is the difference between an emergency appointment and an urgent appointment?

_____

_____

_____

6. Explain why a person making an emergency call should never be placed on hold.

_____

_____

_____

Part V: Types of Scheduling

Briefly describe each type of scheduling and list one advantage and one disadvantage of each.

1. Time-specified (stream) scheduling

_____

_____

_____

2. Open office hours

_____

_____

3. Wave scheduling

_____

_____

_____

4. Modified wave scheduling

_____

_____

_____

5. Double booking

_____

_____

_____

6. Grouping procedures

_____

_____

_____

7. Advance booking

_____

_____

_____

Part VI: Special Circumstances

1. How can the medical assistant deal with patients who are consistently late for appointments?

_____

_____

_____

2. How does the medical assistant handle a patient who arrives at the clinic to see the provider but does not have an appointment?

_____

_____

_____

_____

Part VII: The Reception Area

1. Why is the first impression of the provider's office so important to patients?

_____

_____

_____

2. List five items that might be found in the patient reception area.

_____

_____

_____

_____

_____

3. If a computer is provided in the reception area, what cautionary measure should be taken to ensure patients' privacy?

_____

_____

_____

_____

Part VIII: Registration Procedures

1. List six items of demographic information found on a patient information form.

_____

_____

_____

_____

_____

_____

Part IX: Consideration for the Patient's Time

1. Why might a crowded waiting room be a sign of inefficiency rather than the provider's popularity?

_____

_____

_____

2. Delays longer than _____ minutes should be explained to patients, and patients should be allowed to reschedule if they want to do so.

3. No more than _____ _____ _____ patients should be waiting in the reception area at any given time.

4. What feelings do patients often experience when waiting in the provider's office?

_____

_____

_____

_____

Part X: Patient Confidentiality

1. How can the medical assistant help prevent a breach of patient confidentiality by the placement of charts in wall holders?

_____

_____

_____

_____

2. How can the medical assistant help prevent a breach of patient confidentiality while using sign-in sheets?

_____

_____

_____

_____

3. Provide two examples of incidental disclosures.

_____

_____

_____

4. Should the medical assistant ever discipline a disruptive child in the medical office? Why or why not?

_____

_____

_____

Part XI: Evaluating Reception Areas

1. Visit several reception areas in providers' offices, hospitals, and/or clinics or consider your personal provider's office or one you have recently visited. Take note of the appearance and amenities in these facilities. Rate each reception area on a scale of 1 to 10. Total the figures to determine the best reception area.

CASE STUDIES

Case Study 1

Janie Haynes consistently arrives at the clinic between 15 and 45 minutes late. She always has a "good" excuse, but she could make her appointments on time if she had better time management skills. The office manager has mentioned to Paula, the receptionist, that Janie is to be scheduled at 4:45 PM and if she is late, she will not be seen by the provider. Paula books Janie's next three appointments at that time, and Janie actually arrives early. However, on the fourth appointment, Janie arrives at 5:50 PM, and Paula knows that it is her responsibility to tell Janie that she cannot see the provider. How does Paula handle this task? Is there more than one option?

Case Study 2

Jill is the receptionist for Drs. Boles and Bailey, who are psychiatrists. Each week Sara Ables comes to her appointments but brings her two small children, Joey and Julie, ages 8 and 6 years, respectively. When Sara goes back for her appointment, the children are almost uncontrollable in the reception area. Although there are never more than two patients waiting, the kids are a serious disruption in the clinic. When Jill mentioned the problem to Dr. Boles, he said that Sara really needed the sessions and that Jill should try to work with Sara on this issue. What can Jill do to remedy the situation?

WORKPLACE APPLICATION OPTIONS

1. Invite a medical assistant who performs scheduling duties to speak to the class. Determine at least two questions to ask the scheduler in advance. Ask the scheduler to share the most difficult issues he or she faces while performing scheduling duties in the provider's office.

2. Design a registration form for a fictional clinic that includes all information necessary for a new patient. Be creative with logos and fonts. Make the form attractive and easy to understand.

117

PROCEDURE 10-1. MANAGE APPOINTMENT SCHEDULING USING ESTABLISHED PRIORITIES: ESTABLISH THE APPOINTMENT MATRIX

MAERB/CAAHEP COMPETENCIES: VI.P.1.
ABHES COMPETENCIES: 8.d.

TASK: Establish the matrix of the appointment schedule.

CASE STUDY: Dr. Walden takes a lunch break from 11:30 AM to 12:30 PM. She does hospital rounds from 8:00 AM to 9:00 AM Monday through Friday. Dr. Walden prefers to perform all wellness examinations in the morning. Dr. Martin takes a lunch break from 12:30 PM to 1:30 PM. He does hospital rounds from 8:30 AM to 9:30 AM Monday through Friday. Dr. Martin prefers to do all wellness examinations after lunch. Jean Burke, NP, takes a lunch break from 12:00 PM to 1:00 PM. She will be attending a conference from 2:00 PM to 4:00 PM. All providers use catch-up time. Block one appointment interval in the middle of the morning and one appointment interval in the middle of the afternoon for catch-up time for each provider.

EQUIPMENT AND SUPPLIES:
- Appointment book or computer with scheduling software
- Office procedure manual (optional)
- List of providers' availability and preferences
- Black pen, pencil, and highlighters
- Calendar

Standards: Complete the procedure and all critical steps in _____ minutes with a minimum score of 85% within three attempts.

Scoring: Divide the points earned by the total possible points. Failure to perform a critical step, indicated by an asterisk (*), results in an unsatisfactory overall score.

Time began _____ **Time ended** _____ **Total minutes:** _____

Steps	Possible Points	Attempt 1	Attempt 2	Attempt 3
1. Using the calendar, determine when the office is not opened (e.g., holidays, weekends, evenings). Using the appointment book and a black pen, draw an X through the times the office is not opened. Using the scheduling software, block the times the office is not opened.	20	_____	_____	_____
*2. For each provider, identify the times he or she is not available. Using the appointment book, write in the providers' names for each column and then draw an X through their unavailable times. With the scheduling software, select the correct provider and block the times the provider is unavailable. Repeat this process with the software until all the times are blocked.	30	_____	_____	_____
3. Using the office procedure manual or providers' preferences, determine when each provider performs certain types of examinations. In the appointment book, indicate these examinations either by writing the examination times or by highlighting the examination times. Follow the office's procedure on indicating these examination times in the appointment book. When using scheduling software, set up the times for the examinations or use the highlighting feature if available.	20	_____	_____	_____

119

*4. Using the office procedure manual or the list of providers' preferences and availability, identify other times to block on the scheduling matrix. Some providers require catch-up times, and these time slots are blocked. Some medical facilities save appointment times for same-day appointments. When saving appointment times for same-day appointments, make sure to indicate this in the appointment book using pencil, which can be erased, and the patient's information can be entered on the day of the appointment. For the scheduling software, block those times when patients can't be booked and indicate the times for the same-day appointments.

Possible Points: **30** Attempt 1: _____ Attempt 2: _____ Attempt 3: _____

Comments:

Points earned _____ ÷ 100 possible points = **Score** _____ **% Score**

Instructor's signature _____

PROCEDURE 10-2. MANAGE APPOINTMENT SCHEDULING USING ESTABLISHED PRIORITIES: SCHEDULE A NEW PATIENT

MAERB/CAAHEP COMPETENCIES: VI.P.1., VI.A.1., VII.P.3.
ABHES COMPETENCIES: 8.d.

TASK: Schedule a new patient for a first office visit and identify the urgency of the visit using established priorities.

ROLE-PLAY SCENARIO: Patricia Black calls and she is a new patient. She just moved to the area and her asthma has flared up over the last 24 hours, but her albuterol inhaler is empty and she needs a new prescription for it. She states that she is doing okay, but without the albuterol she knows it will get worse within the next few days. According to your screening guidelines, she needs to be seen today and scheduling guidelines indicate she needs a 45-minute appointment.

EQUIPMENT AND SUPPLIES:
- Appointment book or computer with scheduling software
- Scheduling and screening guidelines
- Pencil

Standards: Complete the procedure and all critical steps in _____ minutes with a minimum score of 85% within three attempts.

Scoring: Divide the points earned by the total possible points. Failure to perform a critical step, indicated by an asterisk (*), results in an unsatisfactory overall score.

Time began _____ Time ended _____ Total minutes: _____

Steps	Possible Points	Attempt 1	Attempt 2	Attempt 3
*1. Obtain the patient's demographic information (e.g., full name, birth date, address, and telephone number). Write this information down or enter it into the scheduling software. Verify the information entered or written down.	20	_____	_____	_____
2. Determine whether the patient was referred by another provider.	10	_____	_____	_____
3. Determine the patient's chief complaint and when the first symptoms occurred. Utilize the appointment and screening guidelines as needed.	10	_____	_____	_____
4. Search the appointment book or scheduling software for the first suitable appointment time and an alternate time. Offer the patient a choice of these dates and time. Be open to alternative times if the patient can't make the initial options you gave. Provide additional appointment options as needed.	10	_____	_____	_____
5. Enter the mutually agreeable time into the scheduling software. If you are using an appointment book, enter the patient's name, telephone number, and add NP for new patient.	10	_____	_____	_____
*6. Obtain the patient's insurance information. If new patients are expected to pay at the time of the visit, explain this financial arrangement when the appointment is made.	20	_____	_____	_____

Steps	Possible Points	Attempt 1	Attempt 2	Attempt 3
7. Provide the patient with directions to the office and parking instructions if needed.	10	_____	_____	_____
8. Prior to ending the call, ask if the patient has any questions. Reinforce the date and time of the appointment. Politely and professionally end the call, thanking the patient for calling.	10	_____	_____	_____

Comments:

Points earned _____ ÷ 100 **possible points = Score** _____ **% Score**

Instructor's signature _____

PROCEDURE 10-3. COACH PATIENTS REGARDING OFFICE POLICIES: CREATE THE NEW PATIENT BROCHURE

MAERB/CAAHEP COMPETENCIES: V.P.4.
ABHES COMPETENCIES: 5.c.

TASK: Create a new patient brochure that provides an orientation to the practice and the office's policies and procedures.

ROLE-PLAY SCENARIO: Adam Burns stops by the office and he is interested in establishing with a provider. You need to coach him on the office's information, policies, and procedures.

EQUIPMENT AND SUPPLIES:
- Computer with word processing software
- Office procedure manual (optional)

Standards: Complete the procedure and all critical steps in _____ minutes with a minimum score of 85% within three attempts.

Scoring: Divide the points earned by the total possible points. Failure to perform a critical step, indicated by an asterisk (*), results in an unsatisfactory overall score.

Time began _____ Time ended _____ Total minutes: _____

Steps	Possible Points	Attempt 1	Attempt 2	Attempt 3
*1. Using word processing software, design an informational brochure for patients that provides information about the practice and describes practice procedures. At a minimum, the information should include:	50	_____	_____	_____
a. Description of the practice (type of practice, mission statement)				
b. Location and/or a map of the practice				
c. Contact information (telephone numbers, e-mail and website addresses)				
d. Staff names and credentials				
e. Services offered				
f. Hours of operation				
g. How appointments can be scheduled				
h. Practice policies and procedures (e.g., payment policies, appointment cancelations, medication refill, assistance after hours)				
2. Using the practice's new patient brochure, give a brief summary of the different parts of the brochure including how appointments are scheduled and the practice's policies and procedures.	30	_____	_____	_____

Steps	Possible Points	Attempt 1	Attempt 2	Attempt 3
3. Use active listening skills, by listening to what is said and how the message is said.	10	_____	_____	_____
4. Ask if the person has any questions and listen to the person's questions and needs/wants. Address the questions and clarify any information that is required. Watch and listen for verification of the person's understanding.	10	_____	_____	_____

Comments:

Points earned _____ ÷ 100 possible points = **Score** _____ **% Score**

Instructor's signature _____

PROCEDURE 10-4. MANAGE APPOINTMENT SCHEDULING USING ESTABLISHED PRIORITIES: SCHEDULE AN ESTABLISHED PATIENT

MAERB/CAAHEP COMPETENCIES: VI.P.1., VI.A.1., VII.P.3.
ABHES COMPETENCIES: 8.d.

TASK: Manage the provider's schedule, by scheduling appointments for an established patient and handling rescheduling and a no-show appointment.

ROLE-PLAY SCENARIO: Celia Tapia, DOB 5/18/1970, has just completed her office visit with Dr. Martin and is checking out at your desk. You see that she needs to schedule a follow-up appointment in 2 weeks. The scheduling guidelines indicate a follow-up appointment is 15 minutes long.

EQUIPMENT AND SUPPLIES:
- Appointment book or computer with scheduling software
- Scheduling guidelines
- Pencil, red pen
- Reminder card
- Patient's health record

Standards: Complete the procedure and all critical steps in _____ minutes with a minimum score of 85% within three attempts.

Scoring: Divide the points earned by the total possible points. Failure to perform a critical step, indicated by an asterisk (*), results in an unsatisfactory overall score.

Time began _____ Time ended _____ Total minutes: _____

Steps	Possible Points	Attempt 1	Attempt 2	Attempt 3
*1. Obtain the patient's name and information, purpose of the visit, the provider to be seen, and any scheduling preferences. Using the scheduling software, enter the patient's name and date of birth (DOB). Verify that the correct patient is selected.	20	_____	_____	_____
2. Identify the length of the appointment by using the scheduling guidelines.	10	_____	_____	_____
3. Search the appointment book or scheduling software for the first suitable appointment time and an alternate time. Offer the patient a choice of these dates and times. Be open to alternative times if the patient cannot make the initial options you gave. Provide additional appointment options as needed.	15	_____	_____	_____
4. Using a pencil, write the patient's name and phone number in the appointment book and block out the correct amount of time. Add in any other relevant information per the facility's procedures. With the scheduling software, create the appointment per the facility's guidelines.	15	_____	_____	_____
5. Complete the appointment reminder card and ensure that the date and time on the card match the appointment time in the book or in the software. Give the card to the patient.	10	_____	_____	_____

Steps	Possible Points	Attempt 1	Attempt 2	Attempt 3
Continuation of scenario: **Later that day, Mary Jones calls and needs to reschedule her appointment for the following day at the same time.**	20	_____	_____	_____
*6. When a patient calls to reschedule an appointment, follow steps 1 through 4. When the new appointment is made, make sure to erase the old appointment from the appointment log. With the scheduling software, ensure the old appointment time is removed from the schedule. Repeat the appointment date and time to the patient.				
Continuation of scenario: **Mary Jones no-shows for her follow-up appointment with Dr. Green.**	10	_____	_____	_____
7. In the appointment book using red pen, indicate the patient was a "no show." Using the patient's health record, document that the patient failed to show for the follow-up examination with the provider.				

Comments:

Points earned _____ **÷ 100 possible points = Score** _____ **% Score**

Instructor's signature _____

PROCEDURE 10-5. SCHEDULE A PATIENT PROCEDURE

MAERB/CAAHEP COMPETENCIES: VI.C.3., VI.P.1., VI.P.2., VI.A.1., VII.P.3.
ABHES COMPETENCIES: 8.d.

TASK: Manage the provider's schedule, by scheduling appointments for an established patient and handling rescheduling and a no-show appointment

ROLE-PLAY SCENARIO: Monique Jones has just completed seeing Dr. Walden and is checking out at your desk. She gives you an order from the provider that states she needs to have testing with magnetic resonance imaging (MRI) of her left ankle within 1 week. The radiology department in your facility performs MRI.

EQUIPMENT AND SUPPLIES:
- Provider's order detailing the procedure required
- Computer with order entry software (optional)
- Name, address, and telephone number of facility where procedure will take place
- Patient's demographic and insurance information
- Patient's health record
- Procedure preparation instructions
- Telephone
- Consent form (if required for procedure)

Standards: Complete the procedure and all critical steps in _____ minutes with a minimum score of 85% within three attempts.

Scoring: Divide the points earned by the total possible points. Failure to perform a critical step, indicated by an asterisk (*), results in an unsatisfactory overall score.

Time began _____ **Time ended** _____ **Total minutes:** _____

Steps	Possible Points	Attempt 1	Attempt 2	Attempt 3
*1. Obtain an oral or written order from the provider for the exact procedure to be performed.	20	_____	_____	_____
2. Gather the patient's demographic and insurance information. If using an electronic health record, verify you have the correct patient.	15	_____	_____	_____
3. Determine patient's availability within the time frame provided by the provider for the procedure.	15	_____	_____	_____

Steps	Possible Points	Attempt 1	Attempt 2	Attempt 3
*4. Contact the diagnostic facility and schedule the patient's procedure. If you are using a computerized provider order entry (CPOE) system and your facility performs the procedure, you also need to enter the order using the CPOE system.	20	_____	_____	_____

a. Provide the patient's diagnosis and provider's exact order, including name of procedure and time frame.

b. Establish the date and time for the procedure.

c. Give the patient's name, age, address, telephone number, and insurance information (insurance policy numbers, precertification information, and addresses for filing claims).

d. Determine any special instructions for the patient or special anesthesia requirements.

e. Notify the facility of any urgency for test results.

5. Notify the patient of the arrangements and provide the information in a written format:	10	_____	_____	_____

a. Give the name, address, and telephone number of the diagnostic facility.

b. Specify the date and time to report for the procedure.

c. Give instructions on preparation for the test (e.g., eating restrictions, fluids, medications, enemas).

d. If using another facility, the patient will need to bring a form of picture identification and the insurance card.

e. If not using a CPOE system, explain whether the patient needs to pick up orders or whether the order will be sent to the facility in advance.

f. Ask if the patient has any questions and answer the questions.

6. If a consent form is required for the procedure, ensure that the provider has reviewed the form with the patient and that the patient has signed the consent form. A copy of the consent form may be required by the diagnostic facility before the procedure. The consent form should be scanned and uploaded into the electronic health record or placed in the paper record.	10	_____	_____	_____
7. Document the details of the scheduled procedure in the patient's health record. If applicable, create a reminder to check on the procedure results after the appointment date.	10	_____	_____	_____

Comments:

Points earned _____ ÷ 100 possible points = **Score** _____ **% Score**

      Instructor's signature _____

11 Daily Operations in the Ambulatory Care Setting

VOCABULARY REVIEW

Fill in the blanks with the correct vocabulary terms from this chapter.

1. The vendor notified Sally that an item she ordered was _____ and she would receive an e-mail when it was back in stock and ready for shipment.

2. Julie and Jeff inventory the _____ _____ each month to ensure that all the medications and equipment are ready in an emergency.

3. Sarah is considered a(n) _____ _____ because she has a letter stating she can receive Dr. Black's shipments.

4. Mike is _____ because he handles money for the healthcare facility.

5. When Cathy opened a shipment, she looked for the _____ _____, which showed the items in the box.

6. At the end of the day, Daniela has to _____ the examination rooms by replacing the supplies that were used.

7. When Keith needed to purchase printer cartridges, he identified the _____ who sells the brand he needed.

8. Dr. White is not available because she is attending a(n) _____ _____ _____ conference on the latest advancements in orthopedics.

9. Sam switches the phones over to the _____ _____ at the end of the day.

10. Hannah performed a(n) _____ to identify the quantity of supplies available in the department.

11. When preparing for the day, Jessica turns on the stereo, which creates _____ _____ and helps to protect patient confidentiality.

12. When Jack is preparing a purchase order, he needs to identify the _____ _____ _____ for each item so that he orders the correct amount.

13. At the end of the day, Suzanne _____ the equipment in the examination room to remove the debris and reduce the number of microorganisms.

14. Tony knows the printer will _____ over time, and this is used for tax purposes.

15. When Anna sorts the incoming mail, she gives the _____ or billing statements to the business office.

SKILLS AND CONCEPTS

Part I: Matching Exercises
Match when the following activities need to be performed.

a. At the beginning of the day

b. At the end of the day

c. Monthly

1. _____ Follow up on outstanding patient issues and new diagnostic test results

2. _____ Sanitize, disinfect, and sterile equipment and instruments

3. _____ Perform quality control tests

4. _____ Inventory crash carts

5. _____ Activate the alarms

6. _____ Prepare the examination rooms by turning on the lights

7. _____ Switch the phones to the answering service

Part II: Security in the Medical Facility

Read the following scenarios and answer the questions.

1. You are starting a new job as a receptionist. During your orientation, you see the cashbox sitting on the receptionist's desk. Patients arrive, make payments, and the cashbox remains on the desk visible to all and in easy access to the public. How can you safeguard the cashbox when you are the receptionist?

   _____

   _____

   _____

   _____

2. A person staggers up to the reception desk and demands in a loud voice that he needs to be seen immediately for his finger injury. As the patient is talking, he is slurring his orders, he smells of alcohol, and he starts to threaten you if he can't be seen "right now." What strategies can you do to keep yourself and others safe?

   _____

   _____

   _____

   _____

3. The facility's head custodian unlocks the side entrance at 6:00 AM each morning for staff. The door is unsupervised and is labeled "staff only." How might the facility tighten the security during the early morning hours?

   _____

   _____

   _____

   _____

Part III: Equipment and Supplies

1. Describe why the facility should have an inventory list of equipment.

   _____

   _____

2. Describe how the practice's accountant can use the equipment inventory list.

   _____

   _____

130

3. Explain how supervisors can use the equipment inventory list.

_____

_____

4. List seven items that should be documented for each piece of equipment on the inventory list.

_____

_____

_____

_____

_____

_____

5. Explain the purpose of routine maintenance of administrative and clinical equipment.

_____

_____

_____

_____

6. Describe three factors that are taken into consideration when deciding to replace a piece of equipment with a newer model.

_____

_____

_____

_____

7. Explain two reasons that a supervisor or provider may opt to lease a piece of equipment versus buying it.

_____

_____

_____

_____

8. List eight items that should be recorded for each supply in inventory.

_____

_____

_____

_____

_____

_____

_____

_____

131

9. List steps involved in completing an inventory.

_____

_____

_____

_____

_____

_____

_____

10. Describe the usefulness of purchase order numbers for the vendor and the medical facility.

_____

_____

_____

_____

11. On receiving supply deliveries, describe why it is important to check the merchandise as soon as possible.

_____

_____

_____

_____

12. Explain how the packing slip is used when ordered supplies arrive.

_____

_____

_____

_____

Part IV: Handling Mail

1. List five items that affect the postage of an item.

_____

_____

_____

_____

_____

2. List five things that can be done when on the USPS website.

_____

_____

_____

_____

_____

3. Describe Priority Mail.

_____

_____

4. Describe First-Class Mail.

_____

_____

5. When mailing a patient termination letter, explain the benefits of sending it by Certified Mail with Return Receipt.

_____

_____

_____

_____

6. When sorting incoming mail, how is the mail related to patients handled before it is given to the provider?

_____

_____

_____

_____

Part V: Body Mechanics

1. Describe how to safely lift an object.

_____

_____

_____

_____

_____

2. Describe how to get an object that is above your head on a shelf.

_____

_____

_____

Read the case study and answer the questions that follow.

Zachary Brown works for Dr. Tomlinson as a clinical medical assistant. Zach is responsible for clinical medical assistant opening duties. He unlocks supply cabinets, opens examination rooms, turns on the computers in the workstation, and performs the quality control checks on the equipment. When he went to check the temperature of the medication refrigerator and freezer, he found that the refrigerator door had been slightly ajar all night long. The temperature in the refrigerator is 5° F above the maximal temperature. The log was not completed by the medical assistant who closes the door, which is Zach's good friend Sam. Zach knows that Sam has forgotten this in the past and is on warning. Zach is tempted to cover for Sam by changing the morning readings and writing in readings for the prior evening. Should Zach do this? Why or why not?

_____

_____

_____

_____

What is the most professional way to handle this situation?

_____

_____

_____

_____

WORKPLACE APPLICATION OPTIONS

Complete one or more of these activities and, if appropriate, share your results with the class.

1. Set up an interview with an office manager and discuss the cost of running a medical practice from month to month. Describe ways a medical assistant can help decrease the costs.

2. Write a policy and procedure for monitoring temperatures of the refrigerator and freezer that contain medications.

INTERNET ACTIVITY OPTIONS

Complete one or more of these activities and, if appropriate, share your results with the class.

1. Obtain a vaccine name from the instructor and research the storage directions for that medication.

2. Research guidelines for storing vaccines in the refrigerator. Create a sign that provides the key guidelines that must be followed for safe storage.

Name _____ Date _____ Score _____

PROCEDURE 11-1. PERFORM AN INVENTORY WITH DOCUMENTATION: EQUIPMENT INVENTORY

MAERB/CAAHEP COMPETENCIES: VI.P.9.
ABHES COMPETENCIES: 8.e.

TASKS: Perform equipment inventory and document the inventory on the equipment inventory form.

EQUIPMENT AND SUPPLIES:
- Pen
- Administrative and/or clinical equipment
- Purchase information (date, cost, and supplier) and warranty information
- Work Product 11-1 Equipment Inventory Form

Standards: Complete the procedure and all critical steps in _____ minutes with a minimum score of 85% within three attempts.

Scoring: Divide the points earned by the total possible points. Failure to perform a critical step, indicated by an asterisk (*), results in an unsatisfactory overall score.

Time began _____ **Time ended** _____ **Total minutes:** _____

Steps	Possible Points	Attempt 1	Attempt 2	Attempt 3
1. For the equipment to be inventoried, gather the following information for each piece of equipment:	40	_____	_____	_____
• Name of equipment, manufacturer, and serial number				
• Location and facility number if applicable				
• Purchase date, supplier, cost, and warranty information				
*2. Complete the Equipment Inventory Form by adding in the following information for each item inventoried: equipment name, manufacturer, and serial number, location and facility number (if applicable), purchase date/supplier, cost, and warranty information.	50	_____	_____	_____
3. Review the document created. Make any necessary revisions.	10	_____	_____	_____

Comments:

Points earned _____ ÷ 100 possible points = Score _____ % Score

Instructor's signature _____

PROCEDURE 11-2. PERFORM ROUTINE MAINTENANCE OF ADMINISTRATIVE OR CLINICAL EQUIPMENT

MAERB/CAAHEP COMPETENCIES: VI.P.8.
ABHES COMPETENCIES: 8.e.(1)

TASK: Perform routine maintenance of administrative or clinical equipment and document the maintenance on the log.

EQUIPMENT AND SUPPLIES:
- Work Product 11-2 Maintenance Logs
- Administrative or clinical equipment (e.g., thermometer)
- Supplies for routine maintenance (e.g., battery)
- Operation manual if needed
- Pen
- Information regarding the equipment (name, serial number, location, facility number, manufacturer, purchased date, warranty information, frequency of inspections, and service provider)

Standards: Complete the procedure and all critical steps in _____ minutes with a minimum score of 85% within three attempts.

Scoring: Divide the points earned by the total possible points. Failure to perform a critical step, indicated by an asterisk (*), results in an unsatisfactory overall score.

Time began _____ Time ended _____ Total minutes: _____

Steps	Possible Points	Attempt 1	Attempt 2	Attempt 3
1. Gather information on the piece of equipment identified for routine maintenance, including name, serial number, location, facility number, manufacturer, purchased date, warranty information, frequency of inspections, and service provider.	20	_____	_____	_____
*2. Fill in the equipment details on the log.	20	_____	_____	_____
3. To perform the maintenance activities, gather the required supplies. If you are not familiar with the procedure or the required supplies, refer to the operation manual.	10	_____	_____	_____
*4. Perform the maintenance activities as directed in the operation manual. Take any required safety precautions necessary to protect yourself and others.	20	_____	_____	_____
5. Clean up the work area.	10	_____	_____	_____
*6. Using a pen, document the date, time, maintenance activity performed, and your signature on the log.	20	_____	_____	_____

Comments:

Points earned _____ ÷ 100 possible points = **Score** _____ **% Score**

Instructor's signature _____

Name _____ Date _____ Score _____

PROCEDURE 11-3. PERFORM AN INVENTORY WITH DOCUMENTATION: PERFORM AN INVENTORY OF SUPPLIES WHILE USING PROPER BODY MECHANICS

MAERB/CAAHEP COMPETENCIES: VI.P.9., XII.P.3.
ABHES COMPETENCIES: 8.e.

TASKS: Perform a supply inventory using correct body mechanics; document the inventory on the supply inventory form.

EQUIPMENT AND SUPPLIES:
- Pen
- Administrative and/or clinical supplies to be inventoried
- Purchase information (item number, cost, and supplier) for supplies in inventory
- Reorder point and quantity to reorder for each item in inventory
- Work Product 11-3 Supply Inventory Form

Standards: Complete the procedure and all critical steps in _____ minutes with a minimum score of 85% within three attempts.

Scoring: Divide the points earned by the total possible points. Failure to perform a critical step, indicated by an asterisk (*), results in an unsatisfactory overall score.

Time began _____ Time ended _____ Total minutes: _____

Steps	Possible Points	Attempt 1	Attempt 2	Attempt 3
1. For the supplies in inventory, gather the following information for each item: • Name, size, quantity (e.g., each, 100/box) • Item number, supplier's name, cost • Reorder point and quantity to reorder	15	_____	_____	_____
*2. Enter each supply's information on the inventory form, making sure the appropriate data are in the right location.	15	_____	_____	_____
3. Review the document. Make any necessary revisions.	5	_____	_____	_____
*4. Using the supply inventory list, inventory the supplies in the department. Identify how the supply should be counted (e.g., each, by box) and count the number of items in stock.	20	_____	_____	_____
5. Add the number in the appropriate row under the "Stock Available" header.	10	_____	_____	_____
6. Indicate what supplies need to be reordered by checking the appropriate column.	5	_____	_____	_____
7. After counting the item, put the stock back neatly, making sure the oldest stock is in the front.	10	_____	_____	_____
*8. Continue steps 5 through 7 until all supplies are inventoried.	5	_____	_____	_____

Steps	Possible Points	Attempt 1	Attempt 2	Attempt 3
*9. Use proper body mechanics when lifting and moving supplies by maintaining a wide, stable base with your feet. Your feet should be shoulder width apart, and you should have good footing. Bend at the knees, keeping your back straight. Lift smoothly with the major muscles in your arms and legs. Use the same technique when putting the item down.	5	_____	_____	_____
*10. Use proper body mechanics when reaching for an object. Clear away barriers and use a step stool if needed. Your feet should face the object. Avoid twisting or turning when lifting a heavy load.	10	_____	_____	_____

Comments:

Points earned _____ ÷ 100 possible points = **Score** _____ **% Score**

Instructor's signature _____

140

PROCEDURE 11-4. PREPARE A PURCHASE ORDER

TASK: Create an accurate purchase order for supplies.

EQUIPMENT AND SUPPLIES:
- Pen
- Completed Work Product 11-3 Supply Inventory Form or a completed supply inventory list (with item name, size, quantity, item number, supplier's name, reorder point, quantity to reorder, cost, and current stock available) or Work Product 11-4 Completed Inventory Worksheet
- Internet method: computer, internet, and printer
- Catalog method: supply catalog, order form (see Work Product 11-5) and calculator

Standards: Complete the procedure and all critical steps in _____ minutes with a minimum score of 85% within three attempts.

Scoring: Divide the points earned by the total possible points. Failure to perform a critical step, indicated by an asterisk (*), results in an unsatisfactory overall score.

Time began _____ Time ended _____ Total minutes: _____

Steps	Possible Points	Attempt 1	Attempt 2	Attempt 3
1. Review the supply inventory list with the current stock counts and determine what supplies need to be reordered.	20	____	____	____
2. Internet method: Using the internet, find the online store used for ordering the needed supplies.	10	____	____	____
Catalog method: Find a supply catalog that carries the required supplies.		____	____	____
*3. Internet method: Using the search box, type in the item number or description. Verify the item from the search results is what you need to order.	20	____	____	____
Catalog method: Using the catalog, find the item required. Write the information on the order form and calculate the cost using the calculator.		____	____	____
*4. Apply critical thinking skills as you identify the quantity to reorder for that item and order this amount.	15	____	____	____
5. Continue with steps 3 and 4 until all items are ordered.	20	____	____	____
6. When you have finished, verify the contents in your basket/cart or order form. Review the supply inventory list to ensure you have ordered everything that needs to be reordered and ordered the correct quantity of each item.	10			
7. Internet method: Print a copy of the order (in the basket/cart).	5	____	____	____
Catalog method: Complete supplier's information at the top of the order form.		____	____	____

Comments:

Points earned _____ ÷ 100 possible points = Score _____ % Score

Instructor's signature _____

Name: _____ Date: _____

WORK PRODUCT 11-1. EQUIPMENT INVENTORY FORM

To be used with Procedure 11-1

MAERB/CAAHEP COMPETENCIES: VI.P.9.

ABHES COMPETENCIES: 8.e.

Equipment Name	Manufacturer/ Serial Number	Location/Facility Number	Purchase Date/ Supplier	Cost	Warranty Information

Name: _____ Date: _____

WORK PRODUCT 11-2. MAINTENANCE LOGS

To be used with Procedure 11-2

MAERB/CAAHEP COMPETENCIES: VI.P.8.

ABHES COMPETENCIES: 8.e.(1)

Maintenance Log

Equipment: _____ Serial #: _____ Location: _____

Facility #: _____ Manufacturer: _____ Purchased: _____

Warranty Information: _____

Frequency of Inspections: _____

Service Provider: _____

Date	Time	Maintenance Activities	Signature

Maintenance Log

Equipment: _____ Serial #: _____ Location: _____

Facility #: _____ Manufacturer: _____ Purchased: _____

Warranty Information: _____

Frequency of Inspections: _____

Service Provider: _____

Date	Time	Maintenance Activities	Signature

Maintenance Log

Equipment: _____ Serial #: _____ Location: _____

Facility #: _____ Manufacturer: _____ Purchased: _____

Warranty Information: _____

Frequency of Inspections: _____

Service Provider: _____

Date	Time	Maintenance Activities	Signature

Maintenance Log

Equipment: _____ Serial #: _____ Location: _____

Facility #: _____ Manufacturer: _____ Purchased: _____

Warranty Information: _____

Frequency of Inspections: _____

Service Provider: _____

Date	Time	Maintenance Activities	Signature

Name: _____ Date: _____

WORK PRODUCT 11-3. SUPPLY INVENTORY FORM

To be used with Procedure 11-3

MAERB/CAAHEP COMPETENCIES: VI.P.9., XII.P.3.

ABHES COMPETENCIES: 8.e.

Item Name	Size	Quantity	Item Number	Supplier's Name	Reorder Point	Quantity to Reorder	Cost	Stock Available	Order (✓)

Chapter **11   Daily Operations in the Ambulatory Care Setting**

Name: _____ Date: _____

WORK PRODUCT 11-4. COMPLETED INVENTORY WORKSHEET

To be used with Procedure 11-4 (optional)

Note: Since supplies may differ, please complete the following boxes on the table: item number, supplier, and cost information based

Item Name	Size	Quantity	Item Number	Supplier's Name	Reorder Point	Quantity to Reorder	Cost	Stock Available	Order (✓)
Gauze Sponges, non-sterile, 8-ply	2″ × 2″	200/pkg			10	25		9	
Alcohol Prep Pads, sterile, 2 ply		100/box			15	30		12	
Bandages, adhesive strips	¾″ × 3″	100/box			10	35		6	
Dressing, non-adherent, individually wrapped	3″ × 4″	100/box			6	10		8	
Gauze pads, sterile, individually wrapped	4″ × 4″	100/box			25	40		18	
Tape, hypoallergenic paper	1″ × 10 yds	12 rolls/box			10	25		9	
Tape, surgical	1″ × 10 yds	12 rolls/box			10	25		9	
Tape, cloth	1″ × 10 yds	12 rolls/box			10	25		9	

Name: _____ **Date:** _____

WORK PRODUCT 11-5. ORDER FORM

To be used with Procedure 11-4 (optional for catalogue method)

Supplier's Name: _____

Address: _____

Fax number: _____ Website/phone number:_____

Product Number	Description of Product	Qty	Unit	Price/ unit	Cost
			Subtotal		
			Tax (use your local tax rate)		
			Shipping and Handling		
			Final total		

12 The Health Record

VOCABULARY REVIEW

1. Veronica prefers a(n) _____ filing system, in which combinations of letters and numbers are used to identify a file.

2. Julia prefers a(n) _____ filing system, in which the letters of the alphabet are used to identify a file.

3. Paula Ann believes that only a(n) _____ filing system provides patient confidentiality.

4. Dr. Banford uses a(n) _____ file to help him remember that a certain action must be taken on a certain date.

5. Teresa wants to _____ the current software library with programs for making brochures and designing websites.

6. The clinic physician records _____ information when questioning patients about their illness.

7. The clinic physician records _____ information when examining the patient.

8. The office manager is particular about the _____ under which documents are filed because she wants to be able to access information quickly.

9. Dr. Lupez's _____ _____ was irritable bowel syndrome, not colon cancer.

10. José read the memo about the new medical records _____ _____ with interest because his job includes filing.

11. The electronic record that originates from one facility is called the electronic _____ record.

12. The electronic record that originates from more than one facility is called the electronic _____ record.

13. A system that is capable of interacting with another system is said to be _____.

14. The values that determine characteristics or behavior are _____.

15. A conscious, intentional failure or reckless indifference to an obligation is called _____ _____.

16. Meriting condemnation, responsibility, or blame for an act is called _____.

17. A process of electronic data entry of medical practitioner or provider instructions is called _____ _____ _____ _____.

18. The healthcare facility received a _____ _____ _____ that requires them to bring a patient's medical record to court.

19. Dr. Weaver uses _____ for the information needed for the patient's progress notes.

20. Brigitte uses _____ to put Dr. Weaver's information into the electronic health record (EHR).

21. Both the patients and providers have a _____ interest in the information contained in the health record.

22. The 2009 modifications to HIPAA established increasing levels of _____ for violations.

153

23. _____ is never acceptable in health records because it obscures the original entry.

24. Data in EHRs can easily be used for _____ _____ purposes to ensure that all patients receive the highest level of care.

SKILLS AND CONCEPTS

Part I: Filing Medical Records

Using alphabetic filing, place the names below in correct alphabetic order.

1. Cassidy Kay Hale   1. _____
2. Candace Cassidy LeGrand   2. _____
3. Taylor Ann Jackson   3. _____
4. Anton Douglas Conn   4. _____
5. Mitchel Michael Gibson   5. _____
6. Lorienda Gaye Robison   6. _____
7. LaNelle Elva Crumley   7. _____
8. Allison Gaile Yarbrough   8. _____
9. Sarah Kay Haile   9. _____
10. Marie Gracelia Stuart   10. _____
11. Karry Madge Chapmann   11. _____
12. Randi Ann Perez   12. _____
13. Cecelia Gayle Raglan   13. _____
14. Sarah Sue Ragland   14. _____
15. Riley Americus Belk   15. _____
16. Starr Ellen Beall   16. _____
17. Mitchell Thomas Gibson   17. _____
18. George Scott Turner   18. _____
19. Winston Roger Murchison   19. _____
20. Sara Suzelle Montgomery   20. _____
21. Tamika Noelle Frazier   21. _____
22. Alisa Jordan Williams   22. _____
23. Alisha Dawn Chapman   23. _____
24. Bentley James Adams   24. _____
25. Montana Skye Kizer   25. _____
26. Dakota Marie LaRose   26. _____
27. Robbie Sue Metzger   27. _____
28. Thomas Charles Bruin   28. _____
29. Percevial "Butch" Adams   29. _____
30. Carlos Perez Santos   30. _____

Part II: Subjective and Objective Information

Note whether the following information is usually subjective or objective.

Patient's address: _____

Yellowed eyes: _____

Patient's e-mail address: _____

Insurance information: _____

Elevated blood pressure: _____

Bloated stomach: _____

Complaint of headache: _____

Weight of 143 pounds: _____

Bruises on upper arms: _____

Patient's phone number: _____

Part III: Short Answers

1. List five reasons why medical records are kept.

   a. _____

   b. _____

   c. _____

   d. _____

   e. _____

2. Explain the concept of the ownership of medical records.

   _____

   _____

   _____

3. Why might color-coded files be more efficient than an alphabetic filing system?

   _____

   _____

   _____

4. What two major types of patient records are found in a medical office?

   a. _____

   b. _____

5. Describe the difference between an EMR and a practice management system.

   _____

   _____

   _____

6. Identify the categories used for organizing information in a POMR system.

_____

_____

_____

7. Identify the method of organizing information in an SOMR system.

_____

_____

_____

8. Describe the indexing rules for alphabetic filing.

_____

_____

_____

_____

_____

_____

_____

9. Identify equipment and supplies needed to create, maintain, and store health records.

_____

_____

_____

Part IV: Documenting, Changing, and Correcting Medical Records

Correct the following entries as would be done in the health record. Then rewrite the entries correctly. Handwritten corrections are acceptable on these exercises.

1. The correct date of the appointment below was October 12, 20XX.

   10-21-20XX 1330 Patient did not arrive for scheduled appointment. P. Smith, RMA

   _____

2. The patient stated that the chest pain began 2 weeks ago.

   1-31-20XX 10:00 AM Patient complained of chest pain for the past 2 months. No pain noted in arms. No nausea. Desires ECG and blood work to check for heart problems. R. Smithee, CMA

   _____

   _____

   _____

Document the following exercises.

1. Eric Robertson canceled his surgical follow-up appointment today for the third time. Document this information.

   _____

   _____

   _____

   _____

2. Angela Adams called to report that she was not feeling any better since her office visit on Monday. She wants the doctor to call in a refill for her antibiotics. The chart says that she was to return to the clinic on Thursday if she was not feeling better. Today is Monday, and she says she cannot come into the clinic this week. The physician wants to see her before prescribing any other medication. Document this information.

_____

_____

_____

_____

_____

3. Mary Elizabeth Smith called the physician's office to report redness around an injection site. She was in the office 3 hours ago and received an injection of penicillin. She says she also is itching quite a bit around the site and is having trouble breathing. The doctor has left the office for the day. Office policy states that if the physician is out of the office and a patient presents or calls with an emergency, he or she is to be referred to the ER. Document the action that the medical assistant should take.

_____

_____

_____

_____

_____

Part V: Filing Procedures

1. List and explain the five basic filing steps.

a. _____

_____

_____

b. _____

_____

_____

c. _____

_____

_____

d. _____

_____

e. _____

_____

Part VI: Electronic Health Records

1. List five advantages of an EHR system.

a. _____

_____

_____

b. _____

_____

_____

c. _____

_____

_____

d. _____

_____

_____

e. _____

_____

_____

2. List five disadvantages of an EHR system.

a. _____

_____

_____

b. _____

_____

_____

c. _____

_____

_____

d. _____

_____

_____

e. _____

_____

_____

Part VII: American Recovery and Reinvestment Act and HITECH Act

1. By what other name is the American Recovery and Reinvestment Act known?

_____

_____

158

2. What does HITECH stand for?

_____

3. Define *meaningful use*.

_____

_____

_____

4. Define and explain *e-prescribing*.

_____

_____

_____

5. Explain the contents of Subtitle D of the HITECH Act.

_____

_____

_____

6. Define the following terms:

a. Reasonable cause

_____

b. Reasonable diligence

_____

c. Willful neglect

_____

Part VIII: EHR Capabilities

1. What is the approximate cost of implementing an EHR system for a typical physician's office with five physicians?

_____

2. Briefly describe three of the capabilities of an EHR system. Why do you think each capability will enhance patient care?

a. _____

_____

_____

b. _____

_____

_____

c. _____

_____

_____

159

Part IX: The Patient and the EHR

1. Discuss how you would talk with a patient who has expressed legitimate fears about having health information in electronic form. Explain what you would say to the patient and how you would reassure the individual.

_____

_____

_____

Part X: Nonverbal Communication and the EHR

1. List several things to remember when in the examination room with the patient and the electronic device that houses the EMR system. Specifically, what should you do, as the medical assistant, to put the patient at ease?

_____

_____

_____

_____

Part XI: Backup Systems for the EHR

1. List three backup systems for the EHR system in a physician's office.

a. _____

_____

b. _____

_____

c. _____

_____

CASE STUDY

Dr. Adkins and Dr. Brooks want to expand their office to make sure they can take advantage of cutting-edge technology. Their goal is to use electronic equipment to perform as much of the work as possible so that all staff members can keep caring for the patients in the forefront of their mind.

Dr. Adkins is fairly satisfied with the system the clinic has now. However, Dr. Brooks, a "technology geek," wants the newest, greatest, and best electronics in his clinic. The office manager gives Sloan, the medical assistant, the opportunity to research EHR systems to determine which are considered the best of the best.

Research what is available in your local and regional areas, make a brief report about the availabilities, and present it to the class.

1. What new possibilities did you discover in your research?

_____

_____

_____

2. Why do you think many physicians are slow to adopt new technology?

_____

_____

_____

160

3. As a medical assistant, what type of technology would make your duties easier?

_____

_____

_____

_____

WORKPLACE APPLICATION OPTIONS

1. Visit three medical offices and determine the type of filing system that each uses. Ask the receptionist what pros and cons exist for each filing system you encounter. Share this information with the class.

2. Determine whether a local physician's office that uses an EHR system would allow the class to visit, perhaps on an afternoon when patients are not in the clinic. Take a list of at least five questions about using an EHR system. Observe how the system works and watch to see if the employees seem to have more or less of a workload. Watch the interaction of the employees with each other and ask whether they think the system is more of a help or a hindrance as they go about their duties.

INTERNET ACTIVITY OPTIONS

Complete one or more of these activities and, if appropriate, share your results with the class.

1. Use the Internet to investigate various EHR software vendors. Develop a list of positives and a list of negatives about each product found.

2. Use the Internet to investigate color-coding systems for paper-based records. Develop a list of the different systems.

PROCEDURE 12-1. CREATE A PATIENT'S HEALTH RECORD: REGISTER A NEW PATIENT IN THE PRACTICE MANAGEMENT SOFTWARE

MAERB/CAAHEP COMPETENCIES: VI.P.3., VI.P.6., VI.P.7., X.A.2.
ABHES COMPETENCIES: 7.a., 7.b., 8.a.

TASK: Register a new patient in the practice management software, prepare a Notice of Privacy Practices (NPP) form and a Disclosure Authorization form for the new patient, and document in the EHR.

EQUIPMENT AND SUPPLIES:
- Computer with SimChart for the Medical Office or practice management and EHR software
- Completed patient registration form
- Scanner

Standards: Complete the procedure and all critical steps in _____ minutes with a minimum score of 85% within three attempts.

Scoring: Divide the points earned by the total possible points. Failure to perform a critical step, indicated by an asterisk (*), results in an unsatisfactory overall score.

Time began _____ Time ended _____ Total minutes: _____

Steps	Possible Points	Attempt 1	Attempt 2	Attempt 3
1. Obtain new patient's completed registration form. Log into the practice management software.	10	_____	_____	_____
2. Using the patient's last and first names and date of birth, search the database for the patient.	20	_____	_____	_____
*3. If the database does not contain the patient's name, add a new patient and enter the patient's demographics from the completed registration form.	15	_____	_____	_____
*4. Verify that the information entered is correct and that all fields are completed before saving the data.	15	_____	_____	_____
5. Using the EHR software, prepare and print a copy of the Notice of Privacy Practices and a Disclosure Authorization form for the new patient. The Disclosure Authorization form should indicate that the disclosure will be to the patient's insurance company.	15	_____	_____	_____
6. Using the EHR, document that the patient received a copy of the Notice of Privacy Practices and signed the Disclosure Authorization form. Scan the Disclosure Authorization form and upload into the EHR.	15	_____	_____	_____
7. Log out of the software on completion of the procedure.	10	_____	_____	_____

Comments:

Points earned _____ ÷ 100 possible points = Score _____ % Score

Instructor's signature _____

Name _____ Date _____ Score _____

PROCEDURE 12-2. ORGANIZE A PATIENT'S HEALTH RECORD: UPLOAD DOCUMENTS TO THE ELECTRONIC HEALTH RECORD

MAERB/CAAHEP COMPETENCIES: VI.P.4., VI.P.6., VI.P.7.
ABHES COMPETENCIES: 7.a., 7.b., 8.a.

TASK: Scan paper records and upload health record digital files to the EHR.

SCENARIO: New patient XYZ brings in a laboratory report and a radiology report that he would like to be added to his EHR. You need to scan in the original documents and upload them to the EHR.

EQUIPMENT AND SUPPLIES:
- Scanner
- Computer with SimChart for the Medical Office or EHR software
- Patient's laboratory and radiology reports

Standards: Complete the procedure and all critical steps in _____ minutes with a minimum score of 85% within three attempts.

Scoring: Divide the points earned by the total possible points. Failure to perform a critical step, indicated by an asterisk (*), results in an unsatisfactory overall score.

Time began _____ Time ended _____ Total minutes: _____

Steps	Possible Points	Attempt 1	Attempt 2	Attempt 3
1. Obtain the patient's name and date of birth if not on the reports.	10	_____	_____	_____
2. Using a scanner that is connected to the computer, scan each document, creating an individual digital image for each.	20	_____	_____	_____
3. Locate the file of the two scanned images in the computer drive. Open the files to ensure the images are clear.	20	_____	_____	_____
*4. In the EHR, search for the patient, using the patient's last and first name. Verify the patient's date of birth.	25	_____	_____	_____
*5. Locate the window to upload Diagnostic/Lab Results and add a new result. Enter the date of the test. Select the correct type of result. Browse for the image file of the laboratory file and attach the file. Save the information. Select to add a new result and repeat the steps to upload the second report. Verify that both documents were uploaded correctly.	25	_____	_____	_____

Comments:

Points earned _____ ÷ 100 possible points = Score _____ % Score

Instructor's signature _____

PROCEDURE 12-3. CREATE AND ORGANIZE A PATIENT'S PAPER HEALTH RECORD

MAERB/CAAHEP COMPETENCIES: VI.P.3., VI.P.4.
ABHES COMPETENCIES: 7.a., 7.b., 8.a.

TASK: Create a paper health record for a new patient and organize health record documents in a paper health record.

EQUIPMENT AND SUPPLIES:
- End tab file folder
- Completed patient registration form
- Divider sheets with different color labels (4)
- Progress note sheet (1)
- Name label
- Color-coding labels (first two letters of last name and first letter of first name)
- Year label
- Allergy label
- Black pen or computer with word processing software to process labels
- Health record documents (i.e., prior records, laboratory reports)
- Hole puncher

Standards: Complete the procedure and all critical steps in _____ minutes with a minimum score of 85% within three attempts.

Scoring: Divide the points earned by the total possible points. Failure to perform a critical step, indicated by an asterisk (*), results in an unsatisfactory overall score.

Time began _____ Time ended _____ Total minutes: _____

Steps	Possible Points	Attempt 1	Attempt 2	Attempt 3
1. Obtain the patient's first name and last name.	5	____	____	____
2. Neatly write or type the patient's name on the name label. Left-justify the last name, followed by a comma, the first name, middle initial, and a period (e.g., Smith, Mary J.).	5	____	____	____
3. Adhere the name label to the bottom left side of the record tab. When the record is held by the main fold in your left hand, the writing should be easy to read. (For directional purposes, assume the record main fold is on the left and the tab is at the bottom.)	10	____	____	____
4. Put the color-coding labels on the bottom right edge of the folder. Start by placing the first letter of the last name at the farthest right edge. Working left to right, place the second letter of the last name, then the first letter of the first name, and then the year label. The year label should be close to the name label.	10	____	____	____
5. Place the allergy label on the front of the record. If allergies are known, clearly write the allergy on the label in black or blue ink.	10	____	____	____
6. Place the divider labels on the record divider sheets, if they come separately. Ensure that the labels on the divider sheets are staggered so that they do not overlap. Print the name of the section on the front and back of the label. The print should be easy to read when the record is held by the main fold. (Suggested names for dividers: Progress Notes, Laboratory, Correspondence, and Miscellaneous)	10	____	____	____

Steps	Possible Points	Attempt 1	Attempt 2	Attempt 3
7. Using the prongs on the left side of the record, secure the registration form.	10	_____	_____	_____
8. Using the prongs on the right side of the record, secure the index dividers with a progress note sheet under the progress note tab.	10	_____	_____	_____
9. Verify the name and the date of birth on the health records and ensure that they match the information on the health record.	10	_____	_____	_____
*10. Open the prongs on the right side of the record and carefully remove the record to the point where the documents need to be inserted. For the documents being inserted, punch holes in the proper location. Insert into the record and then reassemble the remaining part of the record. Continue to do this until all the documents are filed within the health record.	20	_____	_____	_____

Comments:

Points earned _____ ÷ **100 possible points = Score** _____ **% Score**

Instructor's signature _____

Name _____ Date _____ Score _____

PROCEDURE 12-4. FILE PATIENT HEALTH RECORDS

MAERB/CAAHEP COMPETENCIES: VI.P.5.
ABHES COMPETENCIES: 8.a.

TASK: File patient health records using two different filing systems: the alphabetic system and the numeric system.

SCENARIO: The agency uses the alphabetic system. You need to file health records in the correct location.

EQUIPMENT AND SUPPLIES:
- Paper health records using the alphabetic filing system
- Paper health records using the numeric filing system
- File box(es) or file cabinet

Standards: Complete the procedure and all critical steps in _____ minutes with a minimum score of 85% within three attempts.

Scoring: Divide the points earned by the total possible points. Failure to perform a critical step, indicated by an asterisk (*), results in an unsatisfactory overall score.

Time began _____ **Time ended** _____ **Total minutes:** _____

Steps	Possible Points	Attempt 1	Attempt 2	Attempt 3
1. Using alphabetic guidelines, place the records to be filed in alphabetic order.	20	_____	_____	_____
2. Using the file box or file cabinet, locate the correct spot for the first file.	15	_____	_____	_____
3. Place the health record in the correct location. Continue these filing steps until all the health records are filed.	15	_____	_____	_____
4. Using numeric guidelines, place the records to be filed in numeric order.	20	_____	_____	_____
5. Using the file box or file cabinet, locate the correct spot for the first file.	15	_____	_____	_____
6. Place the health record in the correct location. Continue these filing steps until all the health records are filed.	15	_____	_____	_____

Comments:

Points earned _____ + 100 possible points = Score _____ % Score

Instructor's signature _____

13 Administrative Pharmacology Applications

VOCABULARY REVIEW

Define the following medical terms.

1. Angina pectoris

   _____

2. Bronchodilator

   _____

3. Cirrhosis

   _____

4. Formulary

   _____

5. Hypercholesterolemia

   _____

6. Metabolic alkalosis

   _____

7. Spermicide

   _____

8. Therapeutic range

   _____

9. Benefit-to-risk ratio

   _____

10. Controlled Substances Act

    _____

11. Physical drug dependency

    _____

12. Habituation

    _____

13. Chemical name

_____

14. Trade name

_____

15. PDR

_____

16. USP

_____

17. Systemic effect

_____

18. Subscription

_____

19. Inscription

_____

20. Signature

_____

21. Superscription

_____

22. Identity proofing

_____

23. Antagonism

_____

24. Synergism

_____

25. Potentiation

_____

26. Sublingual

_____

27. Intrathecal injection

_____

28. Diurnal rhythms

_____

Match the following definitions with the correct terms.

_____ 1. Drugs used to treat and cure a disorder; for example, antibiotics cure bacterial infections

_____ 2. Drugs that do not cure a disorder but relieve pain or symptoms related to the condition; for example, use of an antihistamine for allergic symptoms

_____ 3. Drugs that prevent the occurrence of a condition; for example, vaccines prevent the occurrence of specific infectious diseases

_____ 4. Drugs that help determine the cause of a particular health problem; for example, injection of antigen serum for allergy testing

_____ 5. Drugs that provide substances the body needs to maintain health; for example, estrogen replacement therapy for menopausal women and administration of insulin to patients with diabetes

_____ 6. Medications sold without prescription

_____ 7. Drug formulations that are no longer protected by a patent

_____ 8. Term pertaining to a glue-like substance

_____ 9. Term referring to the administration of drugs by injection

_____ 10. An open space, such as within a blood vessel or the intestine, or in the inside of a needle or an examining instrument

_____ 11. Term that refers to an oral medication that is coated to protect the drug against the stomach juices; this design is used to ensure that the medicine is absorbed in the small intestine

a. Prophylactic

b. Therapeutic

c. Replacement

d. Palliative

e. Diagnostic

f. Parenteral

g. Colloidal

h. Generic

i. Enteric coated

j. Over the counter

k. Lumen

SKILLS AND CONCEPTS

For each of the following terms, give an example of that type of drug then define its indications for use, desired effects, side effects, and adverse reactions.

1. Analgesic

   _____

   _____

2. Anesthetic

   _____

   _____

3. Antibiotic

   _____

   _____

4. Antidepressant

   _____

   _____

5. Antihistamine

   _____

   _____

173

6. Antihypertensive

_____

_____

7. Anti-inflammatory

_____

_____

8. Antimigraine

_____

_____

9. Antipruritics

_____

_____

10. Antipsychotics

_____

_____

11. Central nervous system stimulants

_____

_____

12. Diuretics

_____

_____

13. Hypnotics

_____

_____

14. Lipid-lowering agents

_____

_____

15. Oral hypoglycemics

_____

_____

16. Osteoporosis treatment

_____

_____

17. Anticoagulants

_____

_____

18. Monoclonal antibodies

_____

_____

19. Respiratory corticosteroid agents

_____

_____

20. Antifungals

_____

_____

Fill in the blank with DEA (Drug Enforcement Administration), FDA (Food and Drug Administration), or FTC (Federal Trade Commission).

21. The _____ regulates over-the-counter (OTC) drug advertising.

22. The _____, a division of the Department of Health and Human Services, regulates the development and sale of all prescription and OTC drugs.

23. The _____ was established in 1973 as part of the Department of Justice to enforce federal laws on the use of illegal drugs.

24. Every medical practice should have a copy of the Controlled Substances Act regulations. The medical assistant may obtain this list from a regional office of the _____.

25. In addition to approving new drugs for the marketplace, the _____ is also responsible for establishing standards for their purity and strength during the manufacturing process and for ensuring that generic brands are effective and safe.

26. Each physician who prescribes controlled substances or has them on site must register with the _____ for a Controlled Substances Act registration certificate. The physician receives a specific registration number that must be included on all prescriptions for controlled substances.

27. List five specific guidelines for prescription orders for controlled substances.

    a. _____

    b. _____

    c. _____

    d. _____

    e. _____

Indicate which statements are true (T) and which are false (F).

_____ 28. The chemical name represents the drug's exact formula.

_____ 29. The generic drug name is assigned by the manufacturer and is protected by copyright.

_____ 30. Advil is a brand name for the generic drug ibuprofen.

_____ 31. A prescription is an order written by the physician for the compounding or dispensing and administration of drugs to a particular patient.

32. List six factors that can affect a drug's action.

a. _____

b. _____

c. _____

d. _____

e. _____

f. _____

33. Explain the difference between an antitussive medication and an expectorant.

_____

_____

_____

34. Summarize the standards that generic drug manufacturers must meet.

_____

_____

_____

_____

_____

_____

35. Complete the following classification of controlled substances table.

Schedule	Guidelines	Drug Examples
	Have no accepted medical use Have high potential for abuse Are illegal to possess	
II		
	Are accepted for medical use Have less potential for abuse than schedule I or II drugs May cause moderate to low physical dependence or high psychological dependence	
IV	Are accepted for medical use Have low potential for abuse May cause limited physical or psychological dependence	
		Codeine (e.g., in cough medicine), kaolin and pectin, belladonna, Donnagel, Lomotil, ezogabine (Potiga), lacosamide (Vimpat), pregabalin (Lyrica)

36. Complete the following pregnancy risk categories table.

Category of Risk	Category Description
A	
B	
C	
	Drug has proven risk for fetal harm. Human studies show proof of fetal damage.

37. Summarize The Joint Commission's "Do Not Use" abbreviations list.

_____

_____

_____

38. Choose 5 of the top 10 frequently prescribed medications shown in Table 13-7. Using a *Physician's Desk Reference* (PDR) or an online reference that summarizes FDA-approved information, create medication cards for each, including the following information:

   a. Indications for use

   b. Desired effects

   c. Side effects

   d. Adverse reactions

   e. Dosage and administration

   f. Patient education factors

39. Complete the following table of herbal products.

Name	Use	Side Effects and Cautions
	To promote weight loss and antiaging; antioxidant	
Black cohosh	To relieve symptoms of menopause and to treat menstrual irregularities	
Echinacea		
	Laxative; to treat hot flashes and breast pain, to treat arthritis, to prevent high cholesterol and cancer	
Garlic		Some evidence indicates that garlic can slightly lower blood cholesterol levels and may slow development of atherosclerosis.
		Short-term use can safely relieve pregnancy-related nausea and vomiting. Side effects most often reported are gas, bloating, heartburn, and nausea.

Name	Use	Side Effects and Cautions
Asian ginseng		
	To treat asthma, bronchitis, fatigue, and tinnitus; to treat Alzheimer's disease and other types of dementia; to decrease intermittent claudication; to treat sexual dysfunction and multiple sclerosis	
Glucosamine plus chondroitin sulfate	To treat arthritis and joint pain	
Green tea		
	To treat sleep disorders	
Milk thistle (silymarin)	To promote liver health; to treat cirrhosis, chronic hepatitis, and gallbladder disorders; to lower cholesterol; to reduce insulin resistance	
Saw palmetto		
	Traditionally used to treat mental disorders and nerve pain	

CASE STUDIES

Read the case studies and answer the questions that follow.

1. The first patient of the day for Martha, the medical assistant, has some prescriptions that need to be refilled. Look up each of the following drugs in the PDR to become familiar with the drug's indications and possible side effects. Then prepare the prescriptions for the physician's signature:

   a. Crestor 10 mg; take one pill daily. Dispense 90 tablets with three refills.

   b. Atenolol 50 mg; take one and a half pills by mouth every morning. Dispense 1-month supply with one refill.

   c. Xanax 0.5 mg; take one to two tablets at bedtime as needed. Dispense 30 tablets with no refills.

   d. OxyContin 20 mg; take one tablet as needed for relief of pain. Dispense 15 tablets.

```
DEA#: 8543201        John Jones, M.D.    Tel: 917-544-8976
                     108 N. Main St.
                     City, State

Patient _____ DATE _____

ADDRESS _____


Rx:

Disp:

Sig:



Refill _____ Times
Please label ☑    _____
```

```
DEA#: 8543201        John Jones, M.D.    Tel: 917-544-8976
                     108 N. Main St.
                     City, State

Patient _____ DATE _____

ADDRESS _____


Rx:

Disp:

Sig:



Refill _____ Times
Please label ☑    _____
```

```
DEA#: 8543201        John Jones, M.D.    Tel: 917-544-8976
                     108 N. Main St.
                     City, State

Patient _____ DATE _____

ADDRESS _____


Rx:

Disp:

Sig:



Refill _____ Times
Please label ☑   _____
```

```
DEA#: 8543201        John Jones, M.D.    Tel: 917-544-8976
                     108 N. Main St.
                     City, State

Patient _____ DATE _____

ADDRESS _____


Rx:

Disp:

Sig:



Refill _____ Times
Please label ☑   _____
```

2. The physician has recommended OTC medication for treatment of symptoms of the common cold. What types of things should Martha encourage her patients to do when they are choosing an OTC? Summarize three commonly used OTC medications and their possible complications.

_____

_____

_____

3. What types of medication should the medical assistant consider when obtaining a medical history? What information about these medications should be documented in the patient's record?

_____

_____

_____

4. Simon Carmacci, age 78 years, has been prescribed several medications, including Tenormin, Lasix, Lipitor, and Actos. Based on what you have learned about these medications and about the physiologic changes associated with aging, summarize the potential complications of multiple prescriptions for this patient. Should you consider any patient education factors? If so, what are they?

_____

_____

_____

WORKPLACE APPLICATION OPTIONS

Complete one or more of these activities and, if appropriate, share your results with the class.

1. Martha has noticed that the other medical assistants in the office are unsure of the drug classifications for controlled substances. Prepare an educational handout for the office staff to use as a resource. The handout should include the definition of a controlled substance, an explanation of each schedule (I to V), the potential for abuse or addiction, and some examples of drugs in each schedule. Note whether the prescription can be written, faxed, e-prescribed, or oral.

_____

_____

_____

2. The route of administration used for a drug depends on the intended use of the drug. What route of administration would Martha expect for each of the following illnesses or medications (oral, topical, inhaled, sublingual, mucous membrane, or parenteral route)? Why?

   a. Annual flu vaccination

   _____

   b. Bronchodilator for treatment of an acute asthma attack

   _____

   c. Hyperlipidemia

   _____

   d. Nitroglycerin used for angina

   _____

   e. Dermatitis

   _____

   f. Allergic rhinitis

   _____

   g. Insulin

   _____

   h. Tinea pedis

   _____

   i. Conjunctivitis

   _____

Chapter **13** **Administrative Pharmacology Applications**

3. You are working for a practice that has just started implementing e-prescriptions. What are the benefits of electronic prescriptions for the patient and the practice?

_____

_____

_____

_____

4. One of the responsibilities for a certified medical assistant may be to telephone or fax prescription orders into the patient's pharmacy. Explain safe methods for doing so and summarize in your answer the information that must be included for each medication order.

_____

_____

_____

5. You are responsible for disposing of a small amount of a controlled substance: four OxyContin tablets. How can you legally dispose of this medication?

_____

_____

_____

6. The ambulatory care center where you work uses e-prescriptions. Summarize how prescriptions for controlled substances are electronically submitted. Are there any special DEA regulations that must be followed? What is identity proofing?

_____

_____

_____

INTERNET ACTIVITY OPTIONS

Complete one or more of these activities and, if appropriate, share your results with the class.

1. Search the Internet for articles on prescription drug abuse. What are some steps the medical assistant can take to help prevent the abuse of prescription drugs?

2. Using either the PDR or Rx List online service, look up 10 of the most prescribed medications. Make medication cards for these drugs. Be prepared to discuss the indications, side effects, typical dosage levels, route of administration, and patient education factors for these drugs.

3. Search the Internet for information on homeopathic medicine. Refer to the American Institute of Homeopathy at www.homeopathyusa.org. Summarize what you have learned about the homeopathic approach to treating common conditions.

4. Refer to the National Institutes of Health Office of Dietary Supplements (ODS) at http://ods.od.nih.gov/. Click on the ODS videos link and watch the series of five videos about dietary supplements. Summarize what you learned.

HEALTH RECORD ACTIVITIES

1. Mrs. Jones calls the office and states that she wants to discontinue her Diovan 80 mg because she has no prescription coverage. She states, "I feel fine and don't even know why I'm taking this medication!" What patient education can Martha provide to Mrs. Jones to make her understand the importance of continuing her current medication? Document your conversation for the provider's review and recommendations.

_____

_____

_____

2. A patient comes to the office today for a refill of Vicodin ES 7.5/500 mg, one pill every 8 hours as needed with food. After checking the health record, you notice the patient had a prescription written 5 days ago for the same drug and was dispensed 30 pills at that time. Is it too early for this drug to be refilled? Document your interaction with the patient in the health record. What type of information should you include?

_____

_____

_____

3. Facilities who have controlled substances on site must maintain records for each of the drugs. A separate log sheet is required for each controlled container unit. Below is a sample log sheet. Role-play with your partner the documentation required for a container of 20 mg OxyContin tablets; there are 30 tablets in the container, the container ID number is AC41257, and you are to dispense 2 tablets to Amos Constantine for acute back pain.

Controlled Substance: _____

Container Amount: _____

Schedule (II-V): _____

Date	Amount Received	Container ID	Amount Dispensed	Container Balance	Authorized User Initials	Comments

Name _____ Date _____ Score _____

PROCEDURE 13-1. PREPARE A PRESCRIPTION FOR THE PROVIDER'S SIGNATURE

CAAHEP COMPETENCIES: I.C.11., I.P.4.
ABHES COMPETENCIES: 9.f.

TASK: Prepare a prescription for the physician's signature accurately using appropriate abbreviations and the prescription format.

EQUIPMENT AND SUPPLIES:
- Prescription pad
- Drug reference materials if needed
- Black pen
- Patient's record

Standards: Complete the procedure and all critical steps in _____ minutes with a minimum score of 85% in three attempts.

Scoring: Divide the points earned by the total possible points. Failure to perform a critical step, indicated by an asterisk (*), results in an unsatisfactory overall score.

Time began _____ **Time ended** _____ **Total minutes:** _____

Steps	Possible Points	Attempt 1	Attempt 2	Attempt 3
1. Refer to the provider's written order for the prescription. If the provider gives a verbal order to write a prescription, write down the order and review it with the provider for accuracy.	10	_____	_____	_____
*2. If unfamiliar with the medication, look up the drug in a drug reference book (e.g., the PDR) or online reference site.	5	_____	_____	_____
*3. Ask the patient whether he or she is allergic to any drugs.	10	_____	_____	_____
4. Using a prescription pad that has the provider's name, address, and telephone number, begin to transcribe the provider's order. Add the provider's DEA number if the script is for a controlled substance.	10	_____	_____	_____
5. Record the patient's name and address and the date on which the prescription is being written.	10	_____	_____	_____
*6. Next to the Rx, write in legible handwriting the name of the drug (correctly spelled), the dosage form (e.g., tablet, capsule, and so forth, using correct abbreviations), and the strength ordered.	10	_____	_____	_____
*7. On the next line, write "Disp." This is the subscription, which includes directions to the pharmacist on the amount to be dispensed and the form of the drug.	10	_____	_____	_____
*8. Next comes the signature. This includes directions for the patient, such as how and when to take the medicine; it usually is preceded by the symbol Sig.	10	_____	_____	_____
9. The provider has told you the patient can get three refills of the prescription; therefore, this information should be added at the bottom of the prescription on the designated line.	10	_____	_____	_____

Chapter **13** **Administrative Pharmacology Applications**

Steps	Possible Points	Attempt 1	Attempt 2	Attempt 3
*10. The provider must review and sign the prescription before it is given to the patient.	5	_____	_____	_____
11. Document the medication order and any pertinent details as you would in the patient's record. Include patient education and refill information.	10	_____	_____	_____

Documentation in the Medical Record

Telephoning or Faxing a Prescription into the Pharmacy or Transmitting an E-Prescription

Using the steps outlined above, complete the prescription, including the patient's full name and address; the provider's full name and address; the DEA number if the prescription is for a controlled substance (Schedule II drugs must be filled with a written prescription and/or an electronic health record program that is authorized to fill scheduled drugs); and the drug name, strength, dosage form, quantity prescribed, directions for use, and the number of refills (if any) authorized. The provider must review the prescription for accuracy before the medical assistant telephones, faxes, or transmits the prescription to the pharmacy. Document the pharmacy order in the patient's health record as you would for any prescribed drug.

For an e-prescription, access the program for electronic transmission of prescriptions through the patient's record. Complete all of the information required and transmit it to the patient's preferred pharmacy.

Comments:

Points earned _____ ÷ 100 possible points = **Score** _____ **% Score**

Instructor's signature _____

14 Basics of Diagnostic Coding

VOCABULARY REVIEW

Fill in the blanks with the correct vocabulary terms from this chapter.

1. The determination of the nature of a disease, injury, or congenital defect is a(n) _____.

2. _____ is any contact between a patient and a provider of service.

3. _____ is an indication of the presence of an illness.

4. The _____ lists diagnostic terms and related codes in alphabetical order by main terms.

5. _____ are broad sections of the ICD-10-CM coding manual grouped by disease and injuries.

6. Converting oral or written descriptions into alphanumeric designations is called _____.

7. _____ refers to the abbreviations, punctuation, symbols, instructional notations, and related entities that help the medical assistant or coder select an accurate and specific code.

8. The _____ is the information about the diagnosis or diagnoses of the patient that has been extracted from the medical documentation.

9. H&P stands for _____.

10. _____ is the system currently used in the United States for classifying disease to facilitate the collection of statistical data.

11. The SOAP notes system of documentation divides the information into what four areas?

    a. _____

    b. _____

    c. _____

    d. _____

12. The term _____ is found at the etiology code so that the underlying condition is sequenced first followed by the manifestation.

13. ICD-10-CM codes can have up to _____ characters. _____ "x" is used to fill in for positions that don't have characters.

14. _____ are used to map ICD-9-CM codes to the current ICD-10-CM diagnostic codes.

15. To prepare for medical coding, the coder must analyze the patient's health record and _____ the diagnostic statement.

16. The coder must look up codes in the _____ first before assigning the code.

187

17. The coder can use the _____ to code tumors, either malignant or benign.

18. The seventh character in obstetrics coding is used to identify the _____.

SKILLS AND CONCEPTS

Part I: Getting to Know ICD-10-CM Coding

1. Four basic forms of punctuation are used in the Tabular Index. Which of the following is NOT one of the forms of punctuation?

   a. Brackets

   b. Parentheses

   c. Question marks

   d. Braces

   e. Colon

2. Match the following terms.

   a. Main terms

   b. Nonessential modifiers

   c. Subterms

   d. Essential modifiers

   These terms are indented one space to the right under the main term. They change the description of the diagnosis in bold type.

   Appear in bold

   Are found after the main term and are enclosed in parentheses

   Indented one space to the right under the essential modifier

3. Which of the following will **NOT** be a seventh character for an ICD-10-CM code?

   a. Initial encounter

   b. A separate manifestation code

   c. Subsequent encounter

   d. Identify the fetus

4. Which of the following cross reference notes are used to direct the coder to a specific category in the Tabular List?

   a. See note

   b. Includes note

   c. See also note

   d. See category note

Part II: Abstracting the Diagnostic Statement

1. Information pertinent to code selection is culled from a variety of medical documents. Which of the following will NOT contain a diagnostic statement?

   a. Encounter form

   b. Treatment notes

   c. Discharge summary

   d. Operative report

   e. Nurses notes

   f. Radiology report

   g. Pathology report

   h. Laboratory report

188

2. The _____ _____ is the provider's health history evaluation and physical assessment of the patient.

3. The _____ _____ is a statement in the patient's own words that describes why the person is seeking medical attention.

4. The _____ _____ is used for extracting procedure and diagnostic information for patients who underwent surgery.

5. A _____ _____ condition is a disease that manifests over a long period because medical treatment has not resolved it.

6. Coders who have questions on complicated cases can refer to the _____ _____, which is a journal published by the American Hospital Association (AHA).

Part III: Steps of Diagnostic Coding
Please fill in the blanks.

1. Abstract the correct diagnosis from the _____ _____.

2. Use the _____ _____ to look up the diagnosis in the Alphabetic Index.

3. Look up the _____ term in the Alphabetic Index

4. Review the _____ _____ under the main term.

5. Choose the correct _____ based on the _____ statement.

6. Look up the _____ from the Alphabetic Index in the _____.

7. Check for any _____, _____, inclusion notes, _____ notes, or additional _____ symbol.

8. Assign the final _____ diagnosis code.

Part IV: Determining the Main Term and Essential Modifier
Review the following diagnostic statements and determine the main term and essential modifier in the Alphabetic Index.

1. Morgan Smith had an acute myocardial infarction, commonly referred to as a heart attack.

   Main Term: _____   Essential Modifier: _____

2. Georgia Summers went into anaphylactic shock after drinking milk.

   Main Term: _____   Essential Modifier: _____

3. Roger Costen has benign essential hypertension.

   Main Term: _____   Essential Modifier: _____

4. Raul Castro has been diagnosed with iron-deficient anemia.

   Main Term: _____   Essential Modifier: _____

5. Stephanie Thompson has a urinary tract infection.

   Main Term: _____   Essential Modifier: _____

6. Mabel Johnson has rheumatoid arthritis.

   Main Term: _____   Essential Modifier: _____

7. Amanda Smith was diagnosed with multiple sclerosis.

   Main Term: _____   Essential Modifier: _____

8. Hudson Madison suffered a ruptured abdominal aneurysm.

   Main Term: _____   Essential Modifier: _____

9. Don Julius died last week from congestive heart failure.

   Main Term: _____   Essential Modifier: _____

10. Betty White has allergic gastroenteritis.

   Main Term: _____   Essential Modifier: _____

Part V: Coding Exercises—Using the ICD-10-CM Coding Manual

Code the following diagnoses to the highest level of specificity using the ICD-10-CM coding manual.

1. The Smiths' newborn, Jacob, has a birthmark on his neck.

   _____

2. Christopher Epstein suffers with dementia from Parkinson's disease.

   _____

3. Jenny Beaver developed bronchitis over spring break after inhaling carbon dioxide fumes while sitting in a traffic jam. This is her first visit for this condition.

   _____

4. Carolyn Kennedy has experienced dumping syndrome periodically since her gastric bypass surgery.

   _____

5. Robert Hill has experienced pain when he urinates for the past 3 weeks.

   _____

6. Julia Childs has been nauseated for about a week but has no vomiting.

   _____

7. Angela Basset was classified as morbidly obese.

   _____

8. Joseph Jordan was diagnosed with underachievement in school and sent for counseling.

   _____

9. Jessica Lopez was placed in the neonatal ICU because she was diagnosed with transient tachypnea at birth.

   _____

10. Brad Pitt was bitten by a brown recluse spider. This was his first visit for this condition.

   _____

11. Barbara Richland died of rheumatic mitral stenosis.

_____

12. Susan Mitchell had a nasopharyngeal polyp that needs to be removed.

_____

13. Christian Hale, a 3-year-old boy, suffers from croup syndrome.

_____

14. A tetanus toxoid vaccination was administered to a child who stepped on a rusty nail, initial encounter.

_____

15. Mary Carver is in rehabilitation for episodic cocaine dependence.

_____

16. Jonathan Briggs has been diagnosed with attention deficit disorder, without mention of hyperactivity.

_____

17. Camille Davidson has suppurative otitis media in her left ear.

_____

18. Sally Jenson was born with pyloric stenosis and required surgery.

_____

19. Cynthia Henderson has a plantar wart.

_____

20. Eric Lawson was diagnosed with hematospermia.

_____

Part VI: Coding Exercises—Using TruCode Encoder

Code the following diagnoses to the highest level of specificity using TruCode Encoder.

1. Kayla Swift was diagnosed with infectious mononucleosis.

_____

2. Gerald Weaver has osteoarthritis in his right shoulder region.

_____

3. Jeffrey Rush has a personal history of alcoholism.

_____

4. Barry White's alcoholism has caused cirrhosis of the liver without ascites.

_____

5. Frank Emmett had atherosclerosis of the extremities with gangrene.

_____

6. Ginger Chan experienced dermatitis from using facial cosmetics.

_____

Chapter **14** Basics of Diagnostic Coding

7. The Lewises' first child was born with Down syndrome.

_____

8. Lee Anna has experienced painful menstruation during her last three cycles.

_____

9. Gary Stevens was diagnosed with cardiomegaly.

_____

10. Jerry Stein developed Kaposi's sarcoma in his lymph nodes during the final stages of AIDS.

_____

11. Terri Holden attempted suicide, for the second time, using a handful of lithium.

_____

12. Susan French was stung by a jellyfish while swimming off the coast of Mexico.

_____

13. Riley Brown has acute myocarditis.

_____

14. Ordell Thompson has acute esophagitis.

_____

15. Korney Ralphy was diagnosed with systemic lupus erythematosus.

_____

16. Marcia Radson had a skin condition known as bullous pemphigoid, in which blisters form in patches all over her skin.

_____

17. Osteomalacia caused by malnutrition made it impossible for Robbie Hernandez to walk.

_____

18. Henry Casper has oral leukoplakia, which may have been caused by smoking a pipe.

_____

19. Patricia Kielty has had uterine endometriosis for several years and may require a hysterectomy in the future.

_____

20. Robert Bauer dislocated his right shoulder while playing baseball; it was a closed anterior dislocation.

_____

Dr. Rogers has diagnosed Mrs. Felicia Arrant in the past with congestive heart failure and diabetes mellitus type 2 (insulin dependent). She comes to the clinic today complaining of chest pain and has a fever of 101.8°. Code all of these conditions. In which order should these codes be sequenced?

1. _____

2. _____

3. _____

4. _____

5. _____

WORKPLACE APPLICATION

Complete this activity and share your results with the class, if appropriate.

Determine what certifications are available that relate to coding. What are the requirements for obtaining these special certifications? Why might these be beneficial for the medical assistant? Is there a particular certification you are interested in obtaining?

INTERNET ACTIVITIES

Complete one or more of these activities and, if appropriate, share your results with the class.

1. Research the Certified Coding Specialist (CCS) certification by the American Health Information Management Association (AHIMA) and explore opportunities for a career in coding.

2. Locate a job description for a medical coding specialist and compare and contrast the daily duties that coders perform in a hospital and in a medical office setting.

3. Write a report on the importance of coding accurately. Share the information with the class.

4. Research the standards of ethical coding published by AHIMA.org. List and discuss at least three of the standards.

Student Name _____ Date_____

AFFECTIVE COMPETENCY: IX.A.1. USE TACTFUL COMMUNICATION SKILLS WITH MEDICAL PROVIDERS TO ENSURE ACCURATE CODE SELECTION

Explanation: Student must achieve a minimum score of 3 in each category to achieve competency.

Using tactful communication skills means using good manners as you provide truthful sensitive information to another person while considering the person's feelings. Tactful communication skills include verbal and nonverbal communication that shows respect, discretion, compassion, honesty, diplomacy, and courtesy. When you use tactful behaviors you demonstrate professionalism and you preserve relationships by avoiding conflicts and finding common ground.

Many times the medical coder is the expert on the accurate CPT (Current Procedural Terminology) and ICD (International Classification of Diseases) code selections. The highest level of specificity must be used when coding so that appropriate reimbursement can occur. It is not uncommon for the medical coder to interact with providers and assist them in understanding the coding procedure. During these interactions it is crucial that the medical coder provides the information in a professional, organized, and logical manner. Using tactful communication skills is critical to maintaining a healthy working relationship with providers.

Using the following case study, role-play with two peers how you would use tactful communication skills with medical providers to ensure accurate code selection.

You are a new medical coder for the medical practice. You have been on the job for 6 weeks and have been seeing a trend that charges are being downcoded. The required documentation is present in the health records, but the providers have been selecting less specific codes for the appointment types. Your goal today is to explain to the providers the accurate code selection for the appointment types.

Scoring Criteria (1 thru 4)	Excellent Evidence of Learning 4	Adequate Evidence of Learning 3	Limited Evidence of Learning 2	Unacceptable Evidence of Learning 1	Score Attempt 1	Score Attempt 2	Score Attempt 3
Demonstrated tactful verbal communication by being respectful, honest, and courteous.	Student was respectful and courteous in his/her verbal communication while delivering a truthful sensitive message.	Student was respectful and courteous in his/her verbal communication, but the delivery of a truthful sensitive message needs improvement.	Student awkwardly attempted to be respectful and courteous while delivering a truthful sensitive message, but a lot more work is needed on the delivery and/or the tactful behaviors.	Student's response was not respectful or courteous, thus the delivery of the message was unprofessional and lacked tact.			
Displayed tactful nonverbal behaviors when communicating with providers.	Student demonstrated nonverbal behaviors that reflect respect, compassion, diplomacy, and courtesy.	Student demonstrated some nonverbal behaviors that reflect respect, compassion, diplomacy, and courtesy, but a little more improvement is needed.	Student demonstrated limited nonverbal behaviors that reflect respect, compassion, diplomacy, and courtesy, but a lot more improvement is needed.	Student's nonverbal communication was perceived as being awkward, disrespectful, and/or unkind; lacking proper eye contact and/or normal tone of voice.			

194

Instructor Comments:

PROCEDURE 14-1. PERFORM CODING USING THE CURRENT ICD-10-CM MANUAL

MAERB/CAAHEP COMPETENCIES: IX.P.3.
ABHES COMPETENCIES: 8.c.

TASK: Perform accurate diagnosis coding using the ICD-10-CM coding manual.

EQUIPMENT AND SUPPLIES:
- ICD-10-CM manual (current year)
- Encounter form and other relevant health records

Standards: Complete the procedure and all critical steps in _____ minutes with a minimum score of 85% within three attempts.

Scoring: Divide the points earned by the total possible points. Failure to perform a critical step, indicated by an asterisk (*), results in an unsatisfactory overall score.

Time began _____ Time ended _____ Total minutes: _____

Steps	Possible Points	Attempt 1	Attempt 2	Attempt 3
Preparation				
*1. Abstract the diagnostic statement or statements from the encounter form and/or other health records:	10	_____	_____	_____
1) Determine the main terms in the diagnostic statement that describe the patient's condition.				
2) Determine what essential modifiers describe the main term in the diagnostic statement.				
Alphabetic Index				
1. Locate the main terms from the diagnostic statement in the Alphabetic Index.	5	_____	_____	_____
2. Locate the essential modifiers listed under the main terms in the Alphabetic Index.	5	_____	_____	_____
3. Review the conventions and notes in the Alphabetic Index.	5	_____	_____	_____
*4. Choose a tentative code or code range from the Alphabetic Index that matches the diagnostic statement as closely as possible.	10	_____	_____	_____
Tabular List				
1. Look up the codes chosen from the Alphabetic Index in the Tabular List numerically.	5	_____	_____	_____
*2. Review the notes, conventions, and the Official Coding Guidelines associated with the code and code description in the Tabular List.	10	_____	_____	_____
3. Verify the accuracy of the tentative code in the Tabular List.	5	_____	_____	_____

Chapter **14** **Basics of Diagnostic Coding**

Steps	Possible Points	Attempt 1	Attempt 2	Attempt 3
*4. Extend the code to the highest level of specificity (up to the 7th character if required). If a 7th character is required and no codes are present for the 4th, 5th, or 6th characters, it is appropriate to use the dummy placeholder X for these positions.	10	_____	_____	_____
5. Assign the code or codes selected from the Tabular List and document it in the patient's health record.	5	_____	_____	_____

Using the TruCode Encoder Software

Steps	Possible Points	Attempt 1	Attempt 2	Attempt 3
1. Type in the diagnosis from the diagnostic statement into the encoder search box.	5	_____	_____	_____
2. The software will provide a list of main terms that could be related to the diagnosis types in the search box. The coder chooses the main term that represents the diagnostic statement.	5	_____	_____	_____
*3. Based on the main term chosen, a list of essential modifiers is presented. The coder must review the diagnostic statement to ensure that all documented essential modifiers are identified. If the provider does not document an essential modifier, then the coder should not assume that an essential modifier was implied.	10	_____	_____	_____
4. Note the yellow area on the left of the chosen diagnosis. Click on the yellow area and an instructional notes textbox will appear that includes coding guidelines. Follow the coding guidelines to determine the most accurate code.	5	_____	_____	_____
5. Once all of the menus of essential modifiers and subterms have been presented, select the more accurate and specific code based on the diagnostic statement.	5	_____	_____	_____

Comments:

Points earned _____ ÷ 100 possible points = **Score** _____ **% Score**

WORK PRODUCT 14-1. PATIENT ENCOUNTER FORM

Corresponds to PROCEDURE 14-1

MAERB/CAAHEP COMPETENCIES: IX.P.3.
ABHES COMPETENCIES: 8.c.

Please use the following information to complete the encounter form:

Patient: Jana Green

Chart #: 11366184

Date: 03/30/20XX

Put a check mark in the Medicare box.

Put a check mark in the box in front of 99212 and enter a fee of $32.00.

In the "DIAGNOSIS: (IF NOT CHECKED ABOVE)" box put Herpes Zoster (Shingles).

In the BALANCE FIELD put 32.00

YOUR NAME CLINIC
1234 College Avenue
Saint Paul, Minnesota 55316
Phone: (555) 555-2133   Fax: (555) 555-2134

John Porter, MD   Daniel Berg, MD
Roman Jagla, MD   Katherine Olson, PNP
Ann Johnson, MD   Emily Luther, FNP

TELEPHONE:
FAX:

| PATIENT'S NAME | CHART # | DATE | ☐ MEDI-MEDI ☐ MEDICAL
☐ MEDICARE ☐ PRIVATE
☐ SELF PAY ☐ HMO _____ |

✔	CPT/Md	DESCRIPTION	FEE	✔	CPT/Md	DESCRIPTION	FEE	✔	CPT/Md	DESCRIPTION	FEE	✔	CPT/Md	DESCRIPTION	FEE
		OFFICE VISIT—NEW PATIENT				**LAB STUDIES**				**PROCEDURES (continued)**				**INJECTIONS**	
	99202	Focused Ex.			36415	Venipucture			93235	Holter, 24 Hour			90724	Influenza	
	99203	Detailed Ex.			81000	Urinalysis			10061	I & D Abscess Comp.			90732	Pneumococcal	
	99204	Comprehensive Ex.			81003	–w/o Micro			10060	I & D Abscess Simple			J0295	Ampicillin, 1 gr	
	99205	Complex Ex.			84703	HCG (Urine, Pregnancy)			94761	Oximetry w/Exercise			J0696	Rocephine	
		OFFICE VISIT—ESTABLISHED PATIENT			82948	Glucose			93720	Plethysmography			J1030	Depomedrol 40 mg	
	99212	Focused Ex.			82270	Hemoccult			94760	Pulse Oximetry			J2000	Lidocaine 50 cc	
	99213	Expanded Ex.			85023	CBC-diff.			10003	Rem. Sebaceous Cyst			J2175	Demerol	
	99214	Detailed Ex.			85024	CBC w/part diff			11100	Skin Bx			J3360	Valium 5 mg	
	99215	Complex Ex.			85018	Hemoglobin			94010	Spirometry			J1885	Toradol 30 mg IV	
		PREVENTATIVE MEDICINE—NEW PATIENT			88155	Pap Smear			92801	Visual Acuity			J1885	Toradol 60 mg IM	
	99381	< 1 year old			87210	KOH/Saline Wet Mount			17100	Wart Removal			90720	DTP–HIB	
	99382	1–4 year old			87430	Strep Antigen			17101	Wart Removal, 2nd			90746	HEP B—HIB	
	99383	5–11 year old			87060	Throat Culture			17102	Wart Removal, 3–15			90707	MMR	
	99384	12–17 year old			80009	Chem profile			11042	Wound Debrid.			86580	PPD	
	99385	18–39 year old			80061	Lipid profile				**X-RAY**			86580	PPD w/control	
	99386	40–64 year old			82465	Cholesterol			70210	Sinuses			90732	Pneumovax	
	99387	65+ year old			99000	Handling fee			70360	Neck Soft Tissue			90716	Varicella	
		PREVENTATIVE MEDICINE—ESTABLISHED PATIENT				**PROCEDURES**			71010	CXR (PA only)			82607	Vitamin B12 Inj.	
	99391	< 1 year old			92551	Audiometry			71020	Chest 2V			90712	Polio	
	99392	1–4 year old			29705	Cast Removal			72040	C-Spine 2V			90788	TD Adult	
	99393	5–11 year old			2900_	Casting (by location)			72100	Lumbrosacral			95115	Allergy inj., single	
	99394	12–17 year old			92567	Ear Check			73030	Shoulder 2V			95117	Allergry inj., multiple	
	99395	18–39 year old			69210	Ear Wax Rem. 1 2			73070	Elbow 2V					
	99396	40–64 year old			93000	EKG			73120	Hand 2V					
	99397	65+ year old			93005	EKG tracing only			73560	Knee 2V					
					93010	EKG. Int. and Rep			73620	Foot 2V					
					11750	Excision Nail			74000	KUB					
					94375	Flow Volume									

DESCRIPTION   ICD-10-CM

____ Abdominal pain/unspec.......... R10.9	____ Dementia/unspec............... F03	____ MI, acute......................... I21._
____ Abscess........................... L02._	____ Depression, major/unsp...... F32.9	____ MI, old............................ I25.2
____ Allergic reaction............... T78.40_	____ Diab I, no complications...... E10.0	____ Migraine......................... G43.9
____ Alzheimer's disease.......... G30	____ Diab II, no complications...... E11.9	____ Myalgia.......................... M79.1
____ Anemia/unspec.................. D64.9	____ w/kidney complic...... E11.2_	____ Neck pain....................... M54.2
____ Angina/unspec.................. I20.9	____ w/ophthalmic compl...... E11.3_	____ Neuropathy..................... G62.9
____ Anorexia.......................... R63.0	____ w/neurolog compl...... E11.4_	_X_ Nausea........................... R11.1
____ Anxiety/unspec................. F41.9	____ w/circulartory compl..... E11.5_	_X_ Nausea/vomitting............. R11.0
____ Apnea, sleep.................... G47.30	____ Insulin use......................... Z79.4	____ Obesity/unspec................. E66.9
____ Arrhythmia, cardiac........... I49.9	____ Diarrhea/unspec.............. R19.7	____ Osteoarthritis (site).......... M19._
____ Arthritis, rheumatoid.......... M06.9	____ Diverticulitis.................... K57.92	____ Otitis media..................... H66.9_
____ Asthma/unspec................. J45.909	____ Diverticulosis................... K57.90	____ Parkinson's disease.......... G20
____ Atrial fibrillation................ I48.0	____ Dizziness......................... R42	____ Pharyngitis, acute.............. J02.9
____ B-12 deficiency................. E53.8	____ Dysuria........................... R30.0	____ Pleurisy.......................... R09.1
____ Back pain, low.................. M54.5	____ Edema/unspec.................. R60.9	____ Pneumonia...................... J18.9
____ BPH............................... N40	____ Endocarditis..................... I38	____ Pneumonia, viral.............. J12.9
____ Bradycardia/unspec........... R00.1	____ Esophageal reflux K21.0	____ Prostatitis/unspec............. N41.9
____ Broncitis, acute................ J20._	____ Fatigue (lethargy) R53.83	____ PVD............................... I73.9
____ Bronchitis, chronic............ J42	____ FUO.............................. R50.9	____ Radiculopathyp................ M54.1_
____ Bursitis/unspec................. M71.9	____ Gastritis......................... K29.70	____ Rectal bleeding................ K62.5
____ CA, breast....................... C50._	____ Gastroenteritis (colitis)..... K52.9	____ Renal failure.................... N19
____ CA, lung......................... C34._	____ G.I. bleed........................ K92.2	____ Sciatica........................... M54.3_
____ CA, prostate..................... C61	____ Gout/unspec.................... M10.9	____ Shortness of breath.......... R03.02
____ Cellulitis......................... L03._	____ Headache........................ R51	____ Sinusitis, chr./unspec........ J32.9
____ Chest pain/unspec............. R07.9	____ Health exam..................... 200._	____ Syncope......................... R55
____ Cirrhosis, liver/unspec....... K74.60	____ Hematuria/unspec............. R31.9	____ Tachycardia/unspec.......... R00.0
____ Cold, common................... J00	____ Herpes simplex................. B00.9	____ Tachy., supraventric......... I47.1
____ Colitis/unspec................... K51.90	____ Herpes zoster................... B02.9	____ Tedinitix/unspec............... M77.9
____ Confusion........................ R41.0	____ Hiatal hernia..................... K44.9	____ TIA................................ G45.9
____ CHF............................... I50.9	____ HTN (HBP)...................... I10	____ Ulcer, duodenal/unspec...... K26.9
____ Constipation..................... K59.00	____ Hyperlipidemia/unspec....... E78.5	____ Ulcer, gastric/unspec......... K25.9
____ COPD............................. J44.9	____ Hypothyroidism/unspec...... E03.9	____ Ulcer, peptic/unspec.......... K27.9
____ Cough............................. R05	____ Impotence....................... N52._	____ URI/unspec...................... J06.9
____ Crohn's disease/unspec...... K50.90	____ Influenza, respiratory......... J10.1	____ UTI................................ N39.0
____ CVA............................... I63.9	____ Insomnia......................... G47.0	____ Vertigo............................ R42
____ Decubitus ulcer................. L89._	____ IBS, diarrhea.................... K58.	____ Weight gain...................... R63.5
____ Dehydration..................... E86.0	____ Lupus, systemic erythim..... M32.9	____ Weight loss...................... R63.4

DIAGNOSIS: (IF NOT CHECKED ABOVE)		TODAY'S FEE	
		AMT. REC'D.	
PROCEDURES: (IF NOT CHECKED ABOVE)	RETURN APPOINTMENT INFORMATION:	REC'D BY: ☐ CASH ☐ CR. CARD ☐ CHECK # _____	
	(DAYS)(WKS.)(MOS.)(PRN)	BALANCE	

200

15 Basics of Procedural Coding

CHAPTER REVIEW

Fill in the blanks with the correct vocabulary terms from this chapter.

1. The CPT code is a five-digit code also known as a _____ code.

2. _____ are found at the beginning of each of the six sections of the CPT coding manual, and Rebecca refers to them often when coding procedures.

3. Category _____ codes are for new experimental procedures or emerging technology.

4. A procedure, service, or diagnosis named after a person is called a(n) _____.

5. The six sections of the CPT manual include:

   a. _____

   b. _____

   c. _____

   d. _____

   e. _____

   f. _____

6. Codes in which the components of a procedure are separated and reported separately are called _____ codes.

7. Code additions that explain circumstances that alter a provided service or provide additional clarification or detail are called _____.

8. The CPT coding manual organizes codes into the Alphabetic Index and the _____.

9. _____ codes provide information on the healthcare facility where services were rendered.

10. The CPT was developed and is maintained by the _____.

11. Describe how to use the most current procedural coding system.

   _____

   _____

   _____

   _____

   _____

   _____

   _____

   _____

   _____

   _____

12. Describe how to use the most current HCPCS level II coding system.

_____

_____

_____

_____

_____

_____

_____

_____

_____

Multiple Choice

_____ 1. The CPT coding manual is updated annually on

    a. January 1   c. October 1

    b. December 31   d. June 1

_____ 2. To find the most accurate code, coders use the following progression:

    a. Categories, subcategories, sections, subsections

    b. Sections, subsections, categories, subcategories

    c. Sections, categories, subsections, subcategories

    d. Subsections, subcategories, sections, categories

_____ 3. The evaluation and management CPT codes are used for insurance reimbursement in the following healthcare settings EXCEPT:

    a. Medical office   c. Nursing home

    b. Weight loss clinic   d. Hospital

_____ 4. The format of HCPCS codes is

    a. All alphanumeric   c. All numeric

    b. First character alpha, then numeric   d. First character numeric, then alpha

Coding Exercises

Code the following procedures with modifiers if appropriate.

CPT Coding

1. Dr. Smith visits Eula Fairbanks, a patient with dementia, in the nursing home for less than 30 minutes and performs an expanded problem-focused examination with MDM of low complexity.

_____

2. Jessica Lundy, a newborn, was admitted to the pediatric critical care unit after her birth, where Dr. Williams provided her initial care.

_____

3. Dr. Partridge participated in a complex, lengthy telephone call lasting 30 minutes, regarding a patient who was scheduled for multiple surgeries.

_____

4. When Terri Anderson was involved in a major car accident, the emergency department physician took a comprehensive history, performed a comprehensive examination, and then made highly complex decisions.

_____

5. Tim Taylor is a new patient with a small cyst on his back. Dr. Young took a problem-focused history, performed a problem-focused examination, and then made straightforward medical decisions.

_____

6. Jim Angelo, an established patient, saw the physician for a minor cut on the back of his hand. The physician spent approximately 10 minutes with Jim.

_____

7. Because Lucille Westerman had multiple health problems, she was admitted for observation after a fainting spell. Dr. Adams took a comprehensive history and performed a comprehensive examination, then made medical decisions of high complexity regarding her care.

_____

8. Dr. Wray saw Tammy Luttrell in the office as a new patient. He took a detailed history and performed a detailed examination, and then made medical decisions of low complexity.

_____

9. Dr. Tompkins visited a new patient at her home and spent about 20 minutes diagnosing and treating her for the flu. A problem-focused history and examination with straightforward MDM was performed.

_____

10. Vera Carpenter was admitted to the hospital for diabetes mellitus, congestive heart failure, and an infection of unknown origin. Dr. Antonetti performed a consultation by doing a detailed history and examination, and MDM of low complexity that took about an hour, including the time spent writing orders in her medical record.

_____

11. Sylvia Julius, an established patient, saw Dr. Bridges for her allergies. The physician took a problem-focused history, performed a problem-focused examination, and made straightforward decisions regarding her care.

_____

12. Anesthesia for vaginal delivery

_____

13. Anesthesia was provided for a brain-dead patient whose organs were being harvested for donation.

_____

14. Laparoscopic biopsy of the left ovary

_____

15. Treatment of a clavicular fracture without manipulation

_____

16. Removal of nasal polyp, right nostril

_____

17. Tonsillectomy and adenoidectomy, younger than 12

_____

Chapter **15** **Basics of Procedural Coding**

18. Left ectopic pregnancy

_____

19. Closed treatment of a coccygeal fracture

_____

20. A radiologic examination of mastoids, two views

_____

21. A chest x-ray examination, four views

_____

22. Magnetic resonance imaging (MRI) of spinal canal

_____

23. Computed tomography (CT) scan of abdomen with contrast material

_____

24. Outpatient kidney imaging with vascular flow

_____

25. Creatine phosphokinase (CPK) total lab test

_____

26. Electrolyte panel

_____

27. Adrenocorticotropic hormone (ACTH) stimulation panel

_____

28. Obstetric panel

_____

29. Total protein urine test

_____

30. Blood alcohol level

_____

31. Acute hepatitis panel

_____

32. Urine pregnancy test

_____

HCPCS Coding
33. Standard wheelchair

_____

34. Gradient compression stocking below knee, 40-50 mm Hg each

_____

35. Above knee, short prosthesis, no knee joint (stubbies), with articulated ankle/foot, dynamically aligned, right leg

_____

36. Disposable contact lens, per lens, one set

_____

37. Polio vaccine, intramuscular route

_____

38. Human papillomavirus (HPV) vaccine, nine types, three-dose schedule, intramuscular route

_____

39. Psychotherapy for crisis; first 60 minutes

_____

40. Ambulance waiting time, 1 hour

_____

CASE STUDIES

Identify all procedures that need to be coded for billing purposes in the following text.

1. Roberta Sleether is a new patient who saw Dr. Morganstern to report feeling tired all the time. She stated that she was exhausted even after a full 8 hours of sleep at night. Roberta said that she did not have much of an appetite and that she had been eating mostly salads and chicken with a bowl of fruit as snacks. She is not overweight and her blood pressure and other vital signs were normal. Dr. Morganstern decided to perform a complete blood count, an electrolyte panel, and a lipid panel. He also ordered a urinalysis, an iron-binding capacity, and a vitamin B_{12} test. The physician asked if she had noticed any blood in her urine or stool, and she denied blood in the urine but did mention she had several episodes of diarrhea. Dr. Morganstern added an occult blood test and a stool culture to check for pathogens. The physician placed Roberta on multivitamin therapy and told her to return in 1 week to discuss her laboratory test results. He spent approximately 30 minutes with Roberta, taking a detailed history and performing a detailed examination, making low-complexity medical decisions. Roberta scheduled her appointment for the following week and left the clinic.

2. **Diagnosis:** Left cheek laceration
   Procedure: Repair left cheek laceration
   After the patient was prepped with local anesthetic to the left cheek area, the cheek was dressed and draped with Betadine. The 1.7 cm chin laceration of the skin was closed with three interrupted 6-0 silk sutures. Gentamicin ointment was applied to the lacerations and a dressing was placed on the left cheek. The patient tolerated the procedure well.
   What is the appropriate CPT code for this procedure?
   Can a modifier be used for this procedure? If so, what would be the most appropriate?
   Because anesthesia was used, can an appropriate anesthesia CPT code be used?

3. **Diagnosis:** Abdominal pain
   Procedure: Esophagogastroduodenoscopy with biopsy
   The patient was premedicated and brought to the endoscopy suite where his throat was anesthetized with Cetacaine spray. He then was placed in the left lateral position and given 2 mg Versed, IV.
   An Olympus gastroscope was advanced into the esophagus, which was well visualized with no significant spasms. Subsequently the scope was advanced into the distal esophagus, which was essentially normal. Then the scope was advanced into the stomach, which showed evidence of erythema and gastritis. The pylorus was intubated and

the duodenal bulb visualized. The duodenal bulb showed severe erythema suggestive of duodenitis. Biopsies of both the duodenum and the stomach were obtained. The scope was withdrawn. The patient tolerated the procedure well.

In the Alphabetic Index, which main term should be used to look up the correct CPT code?

What is the appropriate CPT code for this procedure?

CPT code 43236 is a similar code with submucosal injection. Can this be used if the physician usually performs it, but forgot to document?

WORKPLACE APPLICATIONS

Complete one or more of these activities and share your results with the class, if appropriate.

1. Code the following to develop an encounter form for dermatology procedures that would commonly be performed in the medical office.

CPT Code	Procedure
	Biopsy of skin lesion
	Shaving of a single epidermal lesion with a diameter of 1.2 cm
	Removal of seven skin tags on neck
	Total face dermabrasion
	Removed four warts on left leg

2. Compare the coding procedure using the current year manual with using the TruCode encoder. Which procedure is more time efficient? Which procedure can find the most accurate code? When using the coding manual, how can the anatomy diagrams help coders assign the most accurate code?

INTERNET ACTIVITIES

Complete one or more of these activities and share your results with the class, if appropriate.

1. Research job postings on the internet that relate to medical billing and coding. Review job qualifications and requirements to qualify for the position. Could a graduate from your program apply for this job? If not, what could a graduate do to meet these requirements?

2. Review the necessary elements to code evaluation and management codes. Why is accurate and specific medical documentation required to successfully assign evaluation and management codes?

Student Name _____ Date _____

AFFECTIVE COMPETENCY: IX.A.1. USE TACTFUL COMMUNICATION SKILLS WITH MEDICAL PROVIDERS TO ENSURE ACCURATE CODE SELECTION.

Explanation: Student must achieve a minimum score of 3 in each category to achieve competency.

Using tactful communication skills means using good manners as you provide truthful sensitive information to another person while considering the person's feelings. Tactful communication skills include verbal and nonverbal communication that shows respect, discretion, compassion, honesty, diplomacy, and courtesy. When you use tactful behaviors you demonstrate professionalism and you preserve relationships by avoiding conflicts and finding common ground.

Many times the medical coder is the expert on the accurate CPT (Current Procedural Terminology) and ICD (International Classification of Diseases) code selections. The highest level of specificity must be used when coding so that appropriate reimbursement can occur. It is not uncommon for the medical coder to interact with providers and assist them in understanding the coding procedure. During these interactions it is crucial that the medical coder provides the information in a professional, organized, and logical manner. Using tactful communication skills is critical to maintaining a healthy working relationship with the providers.

Using the following case study, role-play with two peers how you would use tactful communication skills with medical providers to ensure accurate code selection.

You are a new medical coder for the medical practice. You have been on the job for 6 weeks and have been seeing a trend that charges are being downcoded. The required documentation is present in the health records, but the providers have been selecting less specific codes for the appointment types. Your goal today is to explain to the providers the accurate code selection for the appointment types.

Scoring Criteria (1 thru 4)	Excellent Evidence of Learning 4	Adequate Evidence of Learning 3	Limited Evidence of Learning 2	Unacceptable Evidence of Learning 1	Score Attempt 1	Score Attempt 2	Score Attempt 3
Demonstrated tactful verbal communication, by being respectful, honest, and courteous.	Student was respectful and courteous in his/her verbal communication while delivering a truthful sensitive message.	Student was respectful and courteous in his/her verbal communication, but the delivery of a truthful sensitive message needs improvement.	Student awkwardly attempted to be respectful and courteous while delivering a truthful sensitive message, but a lot more work is needed on the delivery and/or the tactful behaviors.	Student's response was not respectful or courteous, thus the delivery of the message was unprofessional and lacked tact.			
Displayed tactful nonverbal behaviors when communicating with providers.	Student demonstrated nonverbal behaviors that reflect respect, compassion, diplomacy, and courtesy.	Student demonstrated some nonverbal behaviors that reflect respect, compassion, diplomacy, and courtesy, but a little more improvement is needed.	Student demonstrated limited nonverbal behaviors that reflect respect, compassion, diplomacy and courtesy, but a lot more improvement is needed.	Student's nonverbal communication was perceived as being awkward, disrespectful, and/or unkind; lacking proper eye contact and/or normal tone of voice.			

Instructor Comments:

PROCEDURE 15-1. PERFORM PROCEDURAL CODING: SURGERY

MAERB/CAAHEP COMPETENCIES: IX.P.1.
ABHES COMPETENCIES: 8.c., 8.e., 8.c.3.

TASK: Use the steps for CPT procedural coding to find the most accurate and specific CPT code.

EQUIPMENT AND SUPPLIES:
- CPT coding manual (current year)
- Surgical report (see Figure 1 in Procedure 15-1)
- TruCode encoder software

Standards: Complete the procedure and all critical steps in _____ minutes with a minimum score of 85% within three attempts.

Scoring: Divide the points earned by the total possible points. Failure to perform a critical step, indicated by an asterisk (*), results in an unsatisfactory overall score.

Time began _____ Time ended _____ Total minutes: _____

Steps	Possible Points	Attempt 1	Attempt 2	Attempt 3
Using a Coding Manual				
1. Abstract the procedures and/or services from the procedural statement in the surgical report.	5	_____	_____	_____
*2. Select the most appropriate main term to begin the search in the Alphabetic Index.	10	_____	_____	_____
3. Once the main term has been located, select the modifying term or terms if needed.	10	_____	_____	_____
4. If the main term cannot be found in the Alphabetic Index, repeat steps 2 and 3 using a different main term, possibly based on the procedural statement.	5	_____	_____	_____
5. Once the CPT code or code range is identified in the Alphabetic Index, disregard any code or code range containing additional descriptions or modifying terms not found in the health record.	10	_____	_____	_____
6. Record the code or code ranges that best match the procedural statements in the surgical report.	5	_____	_____	_____
7. Turn to the Tabular List and find the first code or code range from your search of the Alphabetic Index.	10	_____	_____	_____
*8. Compare the description of the code with the procedural statement in the surgical report. Verify that all or most of the health record documentation matches the code description and that there is no additional information in the code description that is not found in the documentation.	10	_____	_____	_____
*9. Review the coding guidelines and notes for the section, subsection, and code to ensure there are no contraindications for the use of the code. Review the coding conventions and add-on codes if any.	10	_____	_____	_____

Steps	Possible Points	Attempt 1	Attempt 2	Attempt 3
*10. Determine whether a modifier is needed.	10	_____	_____	_____
11. Determine whether a Special Report is required.	10	_____	_____	_____
12. Record the CPT code selected in the health record documentation next to the procedure or service performed and in the appropriate block of the insurance claim form.	5	_____	_____	_____

Using the TruCode Software

1. Abstract the procedures and/or services from the procedural statement in the surgical report.	20	_____	_____	_____
2. Type the main term into the search box and select the CPT. Then click on Show All Results.	10	_____	_____	_____
3. If the main term cannot be found through the search, repeat steps 2 and 3 using a different main term based on the procedural statement.	10	_____	_____	_____
4. Choose the procedure description that is closest to the procedural statement in the surgical report.	30	_____	_____	_____
5. Record the CPT code that best matches the procedural statements in the surgical report in the patient's health record.	30	_____	_____	_____

Comments:

Points earned _____ ÷ **100 possible points = Score** _____ **% Score**

Instructor's signature _____

PROCEDURE 15-2. PERFORM PROCEDURAL CODING: OFFICE VISIT AND IMMUNIZATIONS

MAERB/CAAHEP COMPETENCIES: IX.P.1.
ABHES COMPETENCIES: 8.c., 8.e., 8.c.3.

TASK: Use the steps for CPT Evaluation and Management and Vaccination HCPCS coding to find the most accurate and specific CPT Category I E/M section and HCPCS codes.

EQUIPMENT AND SUPPLIES:
- CPT coding manual (current year)
- HCPCS coding manual (current year)
- Progress Note (see Study Guide Chapter 15) (Figure 1)
- TruCode encoder software

Progress Note for Daniel Miller (DOB 03/12/2012)
04/08/20XX Daniel was seen today for a follow-up visit for his recent case of otitis media in the left ear. The ear infection has completely cleared, and he is now able to receive his hepatitis B vaccine. The office visit involved a problem-focused history, problem-focused examination, and medical decision making of low complexity.

Standards: Complete the procedure and all critical steps in _____ minutes with a minimum score of 85% within three attempts.

Scoring: Divide the points earned by the total possible points. Failure to perform a critical step, indicated by an asterisk (*), results in an unsatisfactory overall score.

Time began _____ Time ended _____ Total minutes: _____

Steps	Possible Points	Attempt 1	Attempt 2	Attempt 3
Part A: CPT E/M Coding				
1. Determine the place of service from the progress note.	5	_____	_____	_____
2. Determine the patient status: new or established.	5	_____	_____	_____
3. Identify the subsection, category, or subcategory of service in the E&M section.	15	_____	_____	_____
4. Determine the level of service.	20	_____	_____	_____
a. Determine the extent of the history obtained.				
b. Determine the extent of the examination performed.				
c. Determine the complexity of medical decision making.				
5. If necessary, compare the medical documentation against the examples in Appendix C (Clinical Examples) of the CPT manual.	5	_____	_____	_____
*6. Select the appropriate level of E&M service code and document it in the patient's health record.	10	_____	_____	_____
Part B: HCPCS Coding with TruCode Encoder Software				
*1. Review the provider documentation.	10	_____	_____	_____

Steps	Possible Points	Attempt 1	Attempt 2	Attempt 3
*2. Type the main term into the search box of the encoder and choose the HCPCS Tabular code set for accurate coding.	10	_____	_____	_____
3. If no modifying term produces an appropriate code or code range, repeat steps 2 and 3 using a different main term classification.	5	_____	_____	_____
*4. Compare the description of the code with the medical documentation.	10	_____	_____	_____
5. Select the appropriate HCPCS immunization code, and document it in the patient's health record.	5	_____	_____	_____

Comments:

Points earned _____ ÷ 100 possible points = **Score** _____ % **Score**

Instructor's signature _____

16 Basics of Health Insurance

Fill in the blanks with the correct vocabulary terms from this chapter.

1. An alphanumeric number issued by the insurance company giving approval of a procedure or service is a(n) _____.

2. The amount payable by an insurance company for a monetary loss to an individual insured by that company, under each coverage, is known as _____.

3. In the United States, healthcare practitioners render services _____ receiving payment.

4. Active duty military personnel, family members of active duty personnel, military retirees and their eligible family members under the age of 65, and the survivors of all uniformed services are covered by _____.

5. The health benefits program run by the Department of Veterans Affairs (VA) that helps eligible beneficiaries pay the cost of specific healthcare services and supplies is the (give acronym) _____.

6. _____ provides periodic payments to replace income when an insured person is unable to work as a result of illness, injury, or disease.

7. The _____ _____ is the date on which insurance coverage begins so that benefits are payable.

8. _____ is the process of confirming health insurance coverage for the patient for the medical service and the date of service.

9. The term for limitations on an insurance contract for which benefits are not payable is _____.

10. A reimbursement model in which the health plan pays the provider's fee for every health insurance claim is called _____.

11. Medicaid and Medicare are examples of _____ plans.

12. A privately sponsored health plan purchased by an employer for their employees is considered a(n) _____ policy.

13. _____ is a third-party system that reimburses a provider when services are rendered for an insured patient.

14. A(n) _____ is a healthcare plan that controls the cost of healthcare delivery by requiring all patients to seek care with a primary care provider to assess if more specialized care is needed.

15. _____ pay for all or a share of the cost of covered services, regardless of which physician, hospital, or other licensed healthcare provider is used. Policyholders of these plans and their dependents choose when and where to get healthcare services.

16. A(n) _____ is health insurance coverage for those who are not covered by their employer group plan.

17. An umbrella term for all healthcare plans that focus on reducing the cost of delivering quality care to patient members in return for scheduled payments and coordinated care through a defined network of primary care physicians and hospitals is _____.

18. A(n) _____ is a healthcare provider who enters into a contract with a specific insurance company or program and agrees to accept the contracted fee schedule.

19. _____ is a process required by some insurance carriers in which the provider obtains authorization to perform certain procedures or services or to refer a patient to a specialist.

20. The payment of a specific sum of money to an insurance company for a list of health insurance benefits is called a(n) _____.

21. The primary care provider who can approve or deny when a patient seeks additional care is referred to as a(n) _____.

22. An insurance term used when a primary care provider wants to send a patient to a specialist is _____.

23. The fee schedule designed to provide national uniform payment of Medicare benefits after adjustment to reflect the differences in practice costs across geographic areas is called the _____.

24. A(n) _____ is funded by an organization with an employee base large enough to enable it to fund its own insurance program.

25. The intermediary and administrator who coordinates patients and providers and processes claims for self-funded plans is called a(n) _____.

26. A government-sponsored program under which authorized dependents of military personnel receive medical care was originally called CHAMPUS but now is called _____.

27. A(n) _____ is a review of individual cases by a committee to make sure services are medically necessary and to study how providers use medical care resources.

28. _____ is an insurance plan for individuals who are injured on the job either by accident or an acquired illness.

29. Health insurance plans pay for health services deemed _____.

30. The _____ was passed in 2010 to assist more Americans in obtaining health insurance.

31. Low- and middle-income Americans can purchase health insurance at a(n) _____ to apply for health insurance and not worry about being denied for a pre-existing condition.

32. There are resources for patients who have questions on health insurance coverage through the Patient Protection and Affordable Care Act, such as _____.

33. Benefits cover the _____, or the amount that should be paid to the healthcare provider for services rendered.

34. Patients have a higher financial responsibility when they access care that is _____.

35. _____ are used by many healthcare facility offices to quickly verify eligibility and benefits.

36. When a provider agrees to become a PAR, they also agree to the health insurance plan's _____ for rendered medical services.

37. The _____ is the maximum that third-party payers will pay for a procedure or service.

38. Healthcare providers need to apply to become a _____ through a process called credentialing.

39. The resource-based relative value scale includes the following three parts:

a. _____

b. _____

c. _____

40. _____ are a type of healthcare organization that contracts with various healthcare providers and medical facilities at a reduced payment schedule for their insurance members.

41. A(n) _____ usually takes 3 to 10 working days for review and approval. This type of referral is used when the physician believes that the patient must see a specialist to continue treatment.

42. Prescription drugs are covered by Medicare _____.

SKILLS AND CONCEPTS

Match the following terms and definitions.

_____ Medicaid

_____ Medicare

_____ Medigap

a. A federally sponsored health insurance program for those over 65 years or disabled individuals under 65 years

b. A term sometimes applied to private insurance products that supplement Medicare insurance benefits

c. A federally and state-sponsored health insurance program for the medically indigent

Read the following paragraph and then fill in the blanks.

The medical assistant's tasks related to health insurance processing are initiated when the patient encounters the provider by appointment, as a walk-in, or in the emergency department or hospital. To complete insurance billing and coding properly, the medical assistant must perform the following tasks:

1. Obtain information from the patient and/or the guarantor, including _____ and _____ data.

2. Verify the patient's _____ for insurance payment with the insurance carrier or carriers, as well as insurance _____, exclusions, and whether _____ is required to refer patients to specialists or to perform certain services or procedures, such as surgery or diagnostic tests.

3. Obtain _____ _____ for referral of the patient to a specialist or for special services or procedures that require advance permission.

Match the types of insurance benefits with their description.

_____ Hospitalization

_____ Surgical

_____ Basic medical

_____ Major medical

_____ Disability

_____ Dental care

_____ Vision care

_____ Medicare supplement

_____ Liability insurance

_____ Life insurance

_____ Long-term care insurance

a. A benefits program that offers a variety of options (fee-for-service or managed care plans) that reimburse a portion of a patient's dental expenses and may exclude certain treatments

b. Provides reimbursement for all or a percentage of the cost of refraction, lenses, and frames

c. Helps defray medical costs not covered by Medicare

d. Provides payment of a specified amount upon the insured's death

e. Covers a continuum of broad-range maintenance and health services to chronically ill, disabled, or mentally disabled individuals

f. Pays all or part of a surgeon's or assistant surgeon's fees

g. A form of insurance that insures the beneficiary's earned income against the risk that a disability will make working uncomfortable or impossible and provides weekly or monthly cash benefits

h. Pays all or part of a physician's fee for nonsurgical services, including hospital, home, and office visits

i. Provides protection against especially large medical bills resulting from catastrophic or prolonged illnesses up to a maximum limit, usually after coinsurance and a deductible have been met

j. Pays the cost of all or part of the insured person's hospital room and board and specific hospital services per DRG guidelines

k. Often includes benefits for medical expenses related to traumatic injuries and lost wages payable to individuals who are injured in the insured person's home or in an automobile accident

Answer the following questions.

1. List three advantages of managed care organizations.

    a. _____

    b. _____

    c. _____

2. List three disadvantages of managed care organizations.

    a. _____

    b. _____

    c. _____

3. List two different populations who would qualify for Medicare.

    a. _____

    b. _____

a. List three benefits of the Affordable Care Act.

    a. _____

    b. _____

    c. _____

4. List two different populations who would qualify for Medicaid.

a. _____

b. _____

5. Outline managed care requirements for patient referral.

_____
_____
_____
_____
_____

6. Describe the processes available for the verification of eligibility for services.

_____
_____
_____

CASE STUDY

Survey all class members and determine the various types of insurance coverage that are represented by the students. Have each student call to verify their own health insurance benefits. Choose a medical procedure, such as the flu shot, and have the students call and verify the amounts of coverage for that particular procedure.

WORKPLACE APPLICATIONS

Complete one or more of these activities and share your results with the class, if appropriate.

1. Working in small groups, obtain a quote for health insurance coverage for a family of four from your local health insurance marketplace using the following demographics.

Covered Family Member	Age
Father	38
Mother	35
Son	15
Daughter	10

Use the internet to research health insurance policies and choose three or four from which to obtain quotes.

2. Develop a scenario for a patient with a health maintenance organization (HMO) insurance plan who wants to schedule an appointment with a gastroenterologist for stomach pain. Create a timeline from when the patient first visits the primary care provider (PCP) to when the patient can see the specialist. Include in the timeline the PCP prescribing medication before requesting the referral from the insurance plan and wanting the patient to return in 2 weeks to see how they feel.

Name _____ Date _____ Score _____

PROCEDURE 16-1. INTERPRET INFORMATION ON AN INSURANCE CARD

MAERB/CAAHEP COMPETENCIES: VIII.P.1.
ABHES COMPETENCIES: 8.c.

TASK: Identify essential information on the health insurance ID card in order to confirm co-payment obligations and send accurate health insurance claims for reimbursement.

EQUIPMENT AND SUPPLIES:
- Scanned copy of patient's health insurance ID, both sides
- Scanned copy of patient's state-issued ID card

Standards: Complete the procedure and all critical steps in _____ minutes with a minimum score of 85% within three attempts.

Scoring: Divide the points earned by the total possible points. Failure to perform a critical step, indicated by an asterisk (*), results in an unsatisfactory overall score.

Time began _____ Time ended _____ Total minutes: _____

Steps	Possible Points	Attempt 1	Attempt 2	Attempt 3
1. Review the scanned copy of the patient's health insurance ID card and state-issued ID card in the electronic health record (EHR). If the patient is a minor, then scan a copy of the insured's state-issued ID card.	10	_____	_____	_____
*2. Identify the subscriber on the health insurance ID card with the patient's name. If the patient is different from the insured name on the card, then obtain the relationship with the insured and the insured's sex and date of birth.	25	_____	_____	_____
3. Identify the insurance plan and HMO network, if applicable.	10	_____	_____	_____
4. Identify the insured's policy number and group number.	10	_____	_____	_____
*5. Identify the patient's copayment, which is due before the appointment. Collect the correct amount. For example, if the provider is a general practitioner, then collect the copayment for the PCP.	25	_____	_____	_____
6. On the back of the health insurance ID card, ensure that a customer service phone number and medical claims address is present.	20	_____	_____	_____

Comments:

Points earned _____ ÷ 100 possible points = **Score** _____ **% Score**

Instructor's signature _____

PROCEDURE 16-2. VERIFY ELIGIBILITY OF SERVICES, INCLUDING DOCUMENTATION

MAERB/CAAHEP COMPETENCIES: VIII.P.2.
ABHES COMPETENCIES: 8.c.

TASK: Confirm that the patient's insurance is in effect and determine what benefits are covered and what exclusions, noncovered procedures and services, and precertifications are included or required.

EQUIPMENT AND SUPPLIES:
- Patient health record
- Patient's health insurance identification (ID) card

Standards: Complete the procedure and all critical steps in _____ minutes with a minimum score of 85% within three attempts.

Scoring: Divide the points earned by the total possible points. Failure to perform a critical step, indicated by an asterisk (*), results in an unsatisfactory overall score.

Time began _____ Time ended _____ Total minutes: _____

Steps	Possible Points	Attempt 1	Attempt 2	Attempt 3
1. When a patient calls for an appointment, identify the patient's insurance plan. Ask for information on the patient's ID card, including the subscriber number, the group number, and the phone number for provider services.	25	_____	_____	_____
2. At the time of the appointment, scan both sides of the patient's health insurance ID card(s) and a state-issued ID card.	25	_____	_____	_____
*3. Call the health insurance with the contact number listed on the back of the patient's health insurance ID card, or you can log into the online provider insurance web portal when you have access.	50	_____	_____	_____

Comments:

Points earned _____ ÷ 100 possible points = **Score** _____ **% Score**

       Instructor's signature _____

PROCEDURE 16-3. OBTAIN A REFERRAL WITH DOCUMENTATION

MAERB/CAAHEP COMPETENCIES: VIII.P.3.
ABHES COMPETENCIES: 8.c.

TASK: Obtain a referral from a health plan's provider services desk phone number listed on the back of the patient's health insurance ID card.

EQUIPMENT AND SUPPLIES:
- Patient health record
- Preauthorization form
- Patient's insurance ID card

Standards: Complete the procedure and all critical steps in _____ minutes with a minimum score of 85% within three attempts.

Scoring: Divide the points earned by the total possible points. Failure to perform a critical step, indicated by an asterisk (*), results in an unsatisfactory overall score.

Time began _____ **Time ended** _____ **Total minutes:** _____

Steps	Possible Points	Attempt 1	Attempt 2	Attempt 3
1. Assemble the necessary information, such as the patient ID card, the verification of eligibility, and the online insurance provider web portal login information.	10	_____	_____	_____
2. Examine the patient's health record and determine the service or procedure for which preauthorization is being requested, including the specialist's name and phone number and the reason for the request, if applicable.	10	_____	_____	_____
3. Fill out the preauthorization and/or referral form, providing all information requested.	20	_____	_____	_____
4. Proofread the completed form.	5	_____	_____	_____
5. Attach a copy of the preauthorization submission confirmation into the patient's health record.	5	_____	_____	_____

Comments:

Points earned _____ ÷ **50 possible points = Score** _____ **% Score**

Instructor's signature _____

Name _____ Date _____ Score _____

PROCEDURE 16-4. OBTAIN PREAUTHORIZATION FOR A SURGICAL PROCEDURE WITH DOCUMENTATION

MAERB/CAAHEP COMPETENCIES: VIII.P.3.
ABHES COMPETENCIES: 8.c.

TASK: Obtain preauthorization from a patient's MCO for requested services or procedures with documentation.

EQUIPMENT AND SUPPLIES:
- Patient health record
- Preauthorization form
- Patient's insurance ID card

Standards: Complete the procedure and all critical steps in _____ minutes with a minimum score of 85% within three attempts.

Scoring: Divide the points earned by the total possible points. Failure to perform a critical step, indicated by an asterisk (*), results in an unsatisfactory overall score.

Time began _____ Time ended _____ **Total minutes:** _____

Steps	Possible Points	Attempt 1	Attempt 2	Attempt 3
1. Assemble all necessary information such as the patient ID card and verification of eligibility.	10	_____	_____	_____
2. Examine the patient's health record to determine the procedure for which preauthorization is being requested and assign the appropriate diagnosis and procedural codes for the surgical procedure.	15	_____	_____	_____
3. Fill out the preauthorization form providing all requested information.	20	_____	_____	_____
4. Proofread the completed form.	5	_____	_____	_____
5. Attach a copy of the preauthorization submission confirmation into the patient's health record.	5	_____	_____	_____
6. Call the patient to schedule the surgery.	5	_____	_____	_____

Comments:

Points earned _____ ÷ 60 possible points = Score _____ % Score

Instructor's signature _____

Name: _____ Date: _____

WORK PRODUCT 16-1. PREAUTHORIZATION REQUEST FORM

Corresponds to PROCEDURE 16-3 and PROCEDURE 16-4

MAERB/CAAHEP COMPETENCIES: VIII.P.3.
ABHES COMPETENCIES: 8.c.

Preauthorization Request Form

TO BE COMPLETED BY PRIMARY CARE PHYSICIAN OR OUTSIDE PROVIDER

☐ Medicare ☐ Blue Cross/Blue Shield ☐ Tricare ☐ Health Net
☐ Medicaid ☐ Aetna ☐ Cigna ☐ Other
Group No.:_____

Name: (First, Middle Initial, Last)_____ Date:_____
☐ Male ☐ Female Birthdate: _____ Home Telephone Number:_____
Address: _____
Primary Care Physician:_____
Referring Physician:_____
Referred to:_____ Office Telephone number:_____
Address:_____
Diagnosis Code:_____ Diagnosis:_____
Diagnosis Code:_____ Diagnosis:_____
Treatment Plan:_____
Authorization requested for: ☐ Consult only ☐ Treatment Only ☐ Consult/Treatment
☐ Consult/Procedure/Surgery ☐ Diagnostic Tests
Procedure Code:_____ Description:_____
Procedure Code:_____ Description:_____
Place of service: ☐ Office ☐ Outpatient ☐ Inpatient ☐ Other   Number of visits:_____
Facility: _____ Length of stay:_____
List of potential future consultants (i.e., anesthetists, surgical assistants, or medical/surgical):
Physician's Signature:_____

TO BE COMPLETED BY PRIMARY CARE PHYSICIAN

PCP Recommendations:_____ PCP Initials:_____
Date eligibility checked:_____ Effective Date:_____

TO BE COMPLETED BY UTILIZATION MANAGEMENT

Authorized:_____ Auth. No. _____ Not Authorized:_____
Deferred:_____ Modified:_____
Effective Date:_____ Expiration Date:_____

Medical Billing and Reimbursement

VOCABULARY REVIEW

Match the vocabulary term to the correct definition. Write the answer and term on the line next to the correct definition.

Section 1:

1. The process of obtaining the dollar amount approved for a medical procedure or service before the procedure or service is scheduled.
   _____

2. Obtained from health insurance companies and gives the provider approval to render the medical service.
   _____

3. The electronic transfer of data (e.g., electronic claims) between two or more entities. _____

4. A process done prior to claims submission to examine claims for accuracy and completeness. _____

5. A contract between a provider and an insurance company in which the health plan pays a monthly fee per patient while the provider accepts the patient's copay as payment in full for office visits.
   _____

6. The process of obtaining the dollar amount approved for a medical procedure or service before it is scheduled.
   _____

7. Form used by most health insurance payers for claims submitted by providers and suppliers. _____

8. Process by which an insurance carrier allows a provider to submit insurance claims directly to the carrier electronically.
   _____

9. A healthcare provider who has signed a contract with a health insurance plan to accept lower reimbursements for services in return for patient referrals. _____

a. Precertification

b. CMS-1500

c. Direct billing

d. Release of information

e. Participating provider

f. Preauthorization

g. Electronic data interchange

h. Capitation agreements

i. Audit

Section 2:

10. An intermediary that accepts the electronic claim from the provider, reformats the claim to the specifications outlined by the insurance plan, and submits claim. _____

11. An identifier assigned by the Centers for Medicare and Medicaid Services (CMS) that classifies the healthcare provider by license and medical specialties. _____

12. On the EOB where the payer indicates the conditions under which the claim was paid or denied. _____

13. Found on the patient's health insurance ID card and is needed to identify the specific health plan to which the claim should be submitted. _____

14. When provider may be inclined to code to a higher specificity level than the service provided actually involved.
_____

15. Claims with incorrect, missing, or insufficient data.
_____

16. A form that is sent by the insurance company to the provider who submitted the insurance claim with an accompanying check or a document indicating that funds were electronically transferred.
_____

17. Insurance carrier's decision if the tests and treatments indicated by the CPT and HCPCS codes meet the accepted standard of practice to treat the patient's diagnosis indicated by the ICD code.
_____

18. A patient financial responsibility that the subscriber for the policy is contracted per year to pay toward his or her healthcare before the insurance policy reimburses the provider.
_____

19. When a lower specificity level, or more generalized code, is assigned.
_____

20. A policy provision in which the policyholder and the insurance company share the cost of covered medical services in a specified ratio. _____

21. A patient financial responsibility that is due at the time of the office visit. _____

22. Determining whether fraudulent medical billing practices were done with purpose or by accident. _____

a. Transmitter ID

b. Claims clearinghouse

c. Downcoding

d. Explanation of benefits (EOB)

e. National Provider Identifiers (NPIs)

f. Remark codes

g. Medical necessity

h. Dirty claims

i. Copayment

j. Coinsurance

k. Intentional

l. Upcoding

m. Deductible

SKILLS AND CONCEPTS

Part I: Short Answer Questions

1. List four types of information collected when a patient calls to schedule an appointment.

   a. _____

   b. _____

   c. _____

   d. _____

2. At the time of the appointment, what two things are copied or scanned into the computer?

_____

_____

3. Describe how the patient's insurance eligibility is confirmed.

_____

_____

4. The patient's billing record information is often found on the patient registration form. Using Figure 17-1 in the textbook, list the billing information found on the patient registration form.

_____

_____

5. What items should the medical assistant gather when using the paper method to obtain a precertification for a service or procedure? (Tip: see Procedure 17-2.)

_____

_____

6. Describe the processes for precertification using the paper method. What does the medical assistant need to do?

_____

_____

7. Describe the electronic claim form.

_____

_____

8. Describe two ways electronic claims can be submitted.

_____

_____

9. Describe direct billing.

_____

_____

10. Explain the role of a claims clearinghouse.

_____

_____

11. The medical assistant obtained precertification for a procedure. After the procedure was completed, what are six items needed to reference when completing the CMS-1500 Health Insurance Claim Form?

a. _____

b. _____

c. _____

d. _____

e. _____

f. _____

12. Name the three sections of the claim form.

   a. _____

   b. _____

   c. _____

13. Identify information required to file a third-party claim.

   a. What information must be included in Section 1 of the claim form?

      _____

   b. Name 13 pieces of information required in Section 2.

      1) _____

      2) _____

      3) _____

      4) _____

      5) _____

      6) _____

      7) _____

      8) _____

      9) _____

      10) _____

      11) _____

      12) _____

      13) _____

   c. Name 19 pieces of information required in Section 3.

      1) _____

      2) _____

      3) _____

      4) _____

      5) _____

      6) _____

      7) _____

      8) _____

      9) _____

      10) _____

      11) _____

      12) _____

      13) _____

      14) _____

      15) _____

      16) _____

17) _____

18) _____

19) _____

14. In your own words, identify the steps for filing a third-party claim.

_____

_____

_____

15. Differentiate between fraud and abuse.

_____

_____

_____

16. What can be the consequences of coding fraud and abuse?

_____

_____

_____

17. How are changes to the ICD manual made public?

_____

_____

_____

18. Discuss the effects of upcoding and downcoding.

_____

_____

_____

19. How can the medical assistant help prevent delays in reimbursement and denial of payment?

_____

_____

_____

20. What is the purpose of "claim scrubbers"?

_____

_____

_____

21. When a clearinghouse sends a confirmation report, what should the medical biller do?

_____

_____

_____

22. How many business days does it take for the insurance company to process an electronic insurance claim and how many days should you allow?

_____

_____

_____

23. If no further response is received from the insurance company about the claim after a month, what should the medical biller do?

_____

_____

_____

24. To confirm that the claim was received, what information should the medical biller provide to the insurance carrier?

_____

_____

_____

25. Describe the information provided in the explanation of benefits (EOB).

_____

_____

_____

26. When reviewing an EOB, what are two things that need to be verified?

_____

_____

27. What is the equation used to calculate the patient's responsibility as determined by the primary insurance EOB?

_____

_____

_____

28. Once the patient's responsibility has been determined, from the primary insurance EOB, what is the next step for the medical biller to take?

_____

_____

_____

29. What information might be found in the Remarks codes on the EOB?

_____

_____

_____

30. How would a medical biller identify the reason for a rejected claim?

_____

_____

_____

31. What are the two main reasons for denial claims?

_____

_____

32. In your own words, define medical necessity as it applies to diagnostic and procedural coding.

_____

_____

_____

33. Describe a coinsurance of 70/30 ratio.

_____

_____

_____

34. Explain patient financial obligations for services rendered.

_____

_____

_____

Part II: Interpret Information on an Insurance Card

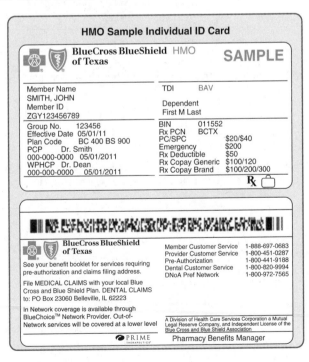

Referring to the information on the ID card, answer the following questions.

1. What is the member's name? _____

2. What is the member's ID number? _____

3. What is the group number? _____

4. Who is the member's primary care provider (PCP)? _____

5. What is the effective date of the plan? _____

6. What is the deductible for prescriptions (Rx)? _____

7. What is the copay for primary care (PC)? _____

8. What number should the patient call if he has a concern? _____

9. What number should you call if you need to get a preauthorization? _____

10. What number should a healthcare professional working with Dr. Smith call if there is a question about the coverage? _____

Part III: Calculating the Coinsurance and Deductible

Use the following information as you answer the following questions.

Patient: Zach Green

Deductible: $750

Coinsurance: 80/20

Patient out-of-pocket expense maximum: $2000

1. During Zach's first visit of the year, he incurred a $500 bill. Who pays this bill?

   _____

   _____

2. During Zach's second visit of the year, he incurred a $450 bill. Describe how much is paid by Zach and the insurance carrier.

   _____

   _____

3. Zach had surgery, which was his third claim of the year. He had a bill of $5,000. Considering the prior visits, what is Zach's typo for this bill and what is the responsibility of the insurance carrier?

   _____

   _____

4. How much is Zach responsible for so far this year considering his first three visits?

   _____

   _____

Part IV: Show Sensitivity When Communicating With Patients Regarding Third-Party Requirements

For this activity, you will role-play a scenario with a peer. Use Procedure 17-1 for this activity.
Scenario: *Ken Thomas saw Jean Burke, NP, for his asthma today. He was prescribed a fluticasone inhaler 220 micrograms (mcg) and a refill on his albuterol inhaler. When Ken stops at the check-out desk to make a follow-up*

appointment, he looks concerned. You inquire how you can help him and he states that he is wondering if his new insurance will pick up the fluticasone inhaler. He further explains that he has used it in the past with great results, but he recently switched insurance plans and he is finding it doesn't have the same coverage as his old plan.

Role play #1: You call the insurance company and discuss the coverage with the insurance carrier's representative. The representative tells you that the fluticasone inhaler is not covered. The representative gives you names of two other inhalers that would be covered.

Role play #2: You must explain to Ken, who is upset with his insurance coverage, that he would have to cover the $250 inhaler.

Clinic information

Walden-Martin Family Medical Clinic, 1234 Anystreet, Anytown, AL 12345

(Phone) 123-123-1234

Insurance ID card information

Policy/ID number: KT4496785

Group number: 55124T

Blue Cross Blue Shield (BC/BS), 1234 Insurance Place, Anytown, AL 12345-1234

For questions, contact Member's Services at 180-012-3111

Part V: Perform Precertification With Documentation

For this activity, you will complete a precertification/prior authorization request form. This activity can be completed using either:

- A paper form (Procedure 17-2 A and Work Product 17-1) or
- SimChart for the Medical Office (Procedure 17-2 B) (Use the Simulation Playground)

Scenario: *You are working with Dr. Julie Walden at Walden-Martin Family Medicine Clinic. Erma Willis (DOB 12/09/1947) was seen for excessive snoring, and Dr. Walden ordered a sleep study. You need to complete a prior authorization/precertification form for the sleep study, which will be conducted by Dr. Jim Sandman. You checked and there is a signed assignment of benefits form on file along with a signed release of information form.*

Insurance Information	Clinic and Provider Information
Aetna	Walden-Martin Family Medical Clinic
1234 Insurance Way	1234 Anystreet
Anytown, AL 12345-1234	Anytown, AL 12345
180-012-3222	Provider: Julie Walden, MD
Member ID Number: EW8884910	Fax: 123-123-5678
Group Number: 66574W	Provider: 123-123-1234
	Provider Contact Name: (your name)

Service Information
Place: Walden-Martin Family Medicine Clinic
Service Requested: Sleep study
Starting Service Date: (1 week from today)
Ending Service Date: (1 week from today)
Service Frequency: one time
ICD-10-CM code: R06.83
CPT-4 code: 95807
Not related to an injury or worker's compensation related.

Part VI: Complete an Insurance Claim Form

For this activity, you will be completing insurance claim forms based on the scenarios. This activity can be completed using either:

- A paper form (Procedure 17-3 A and Work Product 17-2 through 17-5) or
- SimChart for the Medical Office (Procedure 17-3 B) (Use the Simulation Playground. Prior to completing the claim, an encounter needs to be made and a superbill needs to be completed. The ledger is optional, but could also be completed.)

1. Mr. Ken Thomas has suffered from situational depression since the loss of his brother six months ago and has been treated since April 18, 20XX. He was seen on July 23, 20XX by Jean Burke, NP, for treatment of his depression.

Patient Demographics	**Clinic and Provider Information**
Ken H. Thomas (patient and insured)	Walden-Martin Family Medical Clinic
398 Larkin Avenue	1234 Anystreet
Anytown, AL 12345-1234	Anytown, AL 12345
Phone: 123-784-1118	123-123-1234
DOB: 10/25/1961	POS – 04 Independent clinic
SSN: 783-21-2215	Established patient of Jean Burke, NP
HIPAA form on file: Yes – April 18, 20XX	Federal Tax ID# 651249833
Signature on file: Yes – April 18, 20XX	NPI# 1467253823
Insurance Information	
Account Number: 52318	
Blue Cross Blue Shield	
Policy ID Number: KT4496785	
Group Number: 55124T	

Diagnosis	ICD-10-CM Code
Adjustment disorder with mixed anxiety and depressed mood	F43.23

Service	CPT Code	Fee
Est. problem focused OV	99212	$32.00

2. Johnny Parker was seen by Jean Burke, NP, on June 21, 20XX for a well-child check. He had been complaining of a fever and sore throat. The rapid strep test came back positive. Jean Burke, NP gave him a prescription for amoxicillin.

Patient Demographics	**Clinic and Provider Information**
Johnny Parker	Walden-Martin Family Medical Clinic
91 Poplar Street	1234 Anystreet
Anytown, AL 12345-1234	Anytown, AL 12345
Phone: 123-323-6746	123-123-1234
DOB: 06/15/2010	POS – 04 Independent clinic
SSN: 646-81-4747	Established patient of Jean Burke, NP
	Federal Tax ID# 651249833
	NPI# 1467253823
Guarantor Information	**Insurance Information**
Lisa Parker (mother)	Blue Cross Blue Shield
DOB: 10/30/1985	Policy/ID Number: CJ2341783
Address and phone (same as above)	Group Number: 46859J
SSN: 922-11-4747	
Account Number: 74167	
HIPAA form on file: Yes – June 21, 20XX	
Signature on file: Yes – June 21, 20XX	

Diagnosis	ICD-10-CM Code
Encounter for routine child health examination with abnormal findings	Z00.121

Service	CPT Code	Fee
Est. well visit 5–11 y	99393	$65.00
Laboratory – Strep, rapid	87880	$21.00

3. Mr. Walter Biller had an appointment with Dr. Walden on November 16, 20XX. He came in for an influenza vaccine, and while he was there wanted Dr. Walden to look at his ear because he was having problems hearing. His right ear canal was impacted with cerumen, which was irrigated and the cerumen was removed during the visit.

Patient Demographics	Clinic and Provider Information
Walter B. Biller (patient and insured) 87 Willoughby Lane Anytown, AL 12345-1234 Phone: 123-237-3748 DOB: 01/04/1970 SSN: 285-77-7796 HIPAA form on file: Yes – March 19, 20XX Signature on file: Yes – March 19, 20XX	Walden-Martin Family Medical Clinic 1234 Anystreet Anytown, AL 12345 123-123-1234 POS – 04 Independent clinic Established patient of Julie Walden, MD Federal Tax ID# 651249831 NPI# 1467253823
Insurance Information Account Number: 16611 Aetna Policy/ID Number: CH8327753 Group Number: 33347H	

Diagnosis:	ICD-10-CM code
Impacted cerumen, right ear	H61.21

Service	CPT Code	Fee
Est. minimal OV	99211	$24.00
Cerumen removal	69210	$46.00
Vaccine – Flu, 3 Y+	90658	$24.00
Preventive - Flu Administration	G0008	$7.00

4. Aaron Jackson was seen by Dr. Walden on October 12, 20XX for a well-child check. He was delayed completing his immunizations for his age and received the remaining vaccines (MMR and varicella) during the visit.

Patient Demographics	Clinic and Provider Information
Aaron Jackson 555 McArthur Ave Anytown, AL 12345-1234 Phone: 123-814-7844 DOB: 10/17/2011 SSN: 164-72-4618	Walden-Martin Family Medical Clinic 1234 Anystreet Anytown, AL 12345 123-123-1234 POS – 04 Independent clinic Established patient of Julie Walden, MD Federal Tax ID# 651249831 NPI# 1467253823
Guarantor Information Patricia Jackson (mother) DOB: 06/07/1976 Address and phone (same as above) SSN: 190-71-2356 HIPAA form on file: Yes – March 1, 20XX Signature on file: Yes – March 1, 20XX	**Insurance Information** Account Number: 64207 Blue Cross Blue Shield Policy/ID Number: AJ3035489 Group Number: 986541

Diagnosis:		ICD-10-CM code
Encounter for routine child health examination without abnormal findings		Z00.129

Service	CPT Code	Fee
Est. well visit 5–11 y	99393	$65.00
Vaccine, MMR	90707	$59.50
Vaccine, varicella	90716	$32.00
Imm admin, one	90471	$10.00
Imm admin, each add'l	90472	$10.00

Part VII: Use Medical Necessity Guidelines

For this activity, you will complete a claim form showing the accurate information related to the encounter. This activity can be completed using either:

- A paper form (Procedure 17-4 and Work Product 17-6) or
- SimChart for the Medical Office (Procedure 17-4). (Use the Simulation Playground. Prior to completing the claim, an encounter needs to be made and a superbill needs to be completed. The ledger is optional, but could also be completed.)

Scenario: *You are working at Walden-Martin Family Medical Clinic, 1234 Anystreet, Anytown, AL 12345 (phone: 123-123-1234). You receive a letter indicating that Medicare has denied the following claim for not being medically necessary:*

Patient: Norma B. Washington   DOB: 08/07/1944   Date of Service: 06/13/20XX

Policy/ID Number: 847744144A

Provider: Julie Walden, MD

ICD: G43.101 (Migraine)   CPT: J3420 (B-12 injection)

You did some research and the information above was the only information sent to Medicare for that encounter. The following information was the correct information for the encounter:

Patient: Norma B. Washington   DOB: 08/01/1944   Date of Service: 06/15/20XX

ICD: G43.101 (Migraine)   CPT: J1885 (Toradol 15 mg - $15.50) and 90772 (Injection, Ther/Proph/Diag - $25.00)
ICD: D51.0 (Vitamin B-12 deficiency anemia)   CPT: J3420 (B-12 injection- $24.00) and 90772 (Injection, Ther/Proph/Diag - $25.00)

To be billed to: Medicare, 1234 Insurance Road, Anytown, AL 12345-1234

Part VIII: Inform a Patient of Financial Obligations for Services Rendered

Role-play the following scenarios with a peer. Use Procedure 17-5 for this activity.

1. **Scenario:** During this role-play, Christi Brown is meeting with you regarding the bill she received in the mail. When she called to make the appointment, she voiced her confusion about the bill, stating she thought her insurance covered everything. You check her record and see that she met her deductible and now needs to pay 20% of the billed amount. She owes $170.

2. **Scenario:** During this role-play, Michael Smith is meeting with you regarding the bill he received in the mail. When he called to make the appointment, he was very concerned because he just was laid off and isn't sure how he will pay the bill. You check his record and see that he met his deductible and now needs to pay 30% of the billed amount. He owes $210.

Sally is the only medical biller in her healthcare agency. One of the two providers orders and performs tests and procedures before getting the needed preauthorizations from the patients' insurance carriers. As a result, the insurance carriers are not covering the claims and the clinic has had to write off thousands of dollars. Discuss how Sally should deal with the situation. How might she display tactful behavior when communicating with the provider about the third-party requirements? How would you deal with this situation if you were in situation like Sally?

WORKPLACE APPLICATION

Select your insurance or an insurance carrier popular in your area. Research the appeal process for denied claims. Describe the process to appeal a claim.

INTERNET ACTIVITIES

Complete one or more of these activities and, if appropriate, share your results with the class.

1. Review the National Uniform Claim Committee website. Summarize the resources available on this website.

2. Research the history of the CMS-1500 claim form. Determine when it was first used and the changes that the form has undergone since its inception. Prepare a report that details these changes, including the most recent modifications to the CMS-1500.

3. Research the most common errors that occur when submitting medical claims. Summarize your findings and discuss how to avoid making these errors in your future career.

Student Name _____ Date _____

AFFECTIVE COMPETENCY VIII.A.2. DISPLAY TACTFUL BEHAVIOR WHEN COMMUNICATING WITH MEDICAL PROVIDERS REGARDING THIRD-PARTY REQUIREMENTS

Explanation: Student must achieve a minimum score of 3 in each category to achieve competency.

Being tactful means using good manners as you provide truthful sensitive information or provide honest critical feedback to another person. Tactful behaviors include showing respect, discretion, compassion, honesty, diplomacy, and courtesy while you deliver a message. Tactful behaviors encompass both nonverbal and verbal communication, including what you say, how you say it, and your body language during the communication. A critical element of being tactful is considering the other person's feelings and reactions as you deliver the information. When you use tactful behaviors, you demonstrate professionalism and you preserve relationships by avoiding conflicts and finding common ground.

Many times the medical biller is the expert on the third-party requirements, and providers rely on the biller to help them understand the requirements. Being tactful with providers as you communicate third-party requirements is critical to your working relationship with the provider and also important in the overall financial scope of the agency. It is crucial to assist the provider in a tactful manner in understanding his or her role in meeting third-party requirements.

Using the following case study, role-play with two peers how you would display tactful behaviors when communicating with medical providers regarding third party requirements.

You are the medical biller for your clinic. The two providers have not been communicating with you regarding procedures that need prior authorization from the insurance carriers. As a result, multiple claims are being denied, and the clinic has had to write off much of the cost. Today, you are talking with the providers, explaining common procedures that require prior authorizations and the process of getting preauthorizations.

Scoring Criteria (1 Thru 4)	Excellent Evidence of Learning 4	Adequate Evidence of Learning 3	Limited Evidence of Learning 2	Unacceptable Evidence of Learning 1	Score Attempt 1	Score Attempt 2	Score Attempt 3
Demonstrated tactful behavior through verbal communication by being respectful, honest, and courteous.	Student was respectful and courteous in his/her verbal communication while delivering a truthful sensitive message.	Student was respectful and courteous in his/her verbal communication, but the delivery of a truthful sensitive message needs improvement.	Student awkwardly attempted to be respectful and courteous while delivering a truthful sensitive message, but a lot more work is needed on the delivery and/or the tactful behaviors.	Student's response was not respectful or courteous, thus the delivery of the message was unprofessional and lacked tact.			
Displayed tactful nonverbal behaviors when communicating with providers.	Student demonstrated nonverbal behaviors that reflect respect, compassion, diplomacy, and courtesy.	Student demonstrated some nonverbal behaviors that reflect respect, compassion, diplomacy, and courtesy, but a little more improvement is needed.	Student demonstrated limited nonverbal behaviors that reflect respect, compassion, diplomacy, and courtesy, but a lot more improvement is needed.	Student's nonverbal communication was perceived as being awkward, disrespectful, and/or unkind; lacking proper eye contact and/or normal tone of voice.			

Instructor Comments

Name _____ Date _____ Score _____

PROCEDURE 17-1. SHOW SENSITIVITY WHEN COMMUNICATING WITH PATIENTS REGARDING THIRD-PARTY REQUIREMENTS

MAERB/CAAHEP COMPETENCIES: VIII.A.1., VIII.A.3.
ABHES COMPETENCIES: 5.c., 8.f.

TASK: Interact professionally with third-party representative and demonstrate sensitivity through verbal and nonverbal communication when discussing third-party requirements with patients.

EQUIPMENT AND SUPPLIES:
- Copy of patient's health insurance ID card
- Prescription for new medication

Standards: Complete the procedure and all critical steps in _____ minutes with a minimum score of 85% within three attempts.

Scoring: Divide the points earned by the total possible points. Failure to perform a critical step, indicated by an asterisk (*), results in an unsatisfactory overall score.

Time began _____ Time ended _____ Total minutes: _____

Steps	Possible Points	Attempt 1	Attempt 2	Attempt 3
1. Gather a copy of the patient's health insurance ID card and the prescription for the new medication.	10	_____	_____	_____
2. Review the insurance card for coverage information and the phone number for providers.	10	_____	_____	_____
3. Call the insurance company and clearly state the patient's information, the patient's question, and the new medication.	10	_____	_____	_____
4. Demonstrate professionalism through verbal communication skills, by stating a respectful, clear, organized message while pronouncing medical terminology and medications correctly.	10	_____	_____	_____
5. Explain to the patient the message from the insurance representative using language that can be understood by the patient.	10	_____	_____	_____
6. Demonstrate sensitivity to the patient by paying attention to and responding appropriately to the patient's nonverbal body language and verbal message.	10	_____	_____	_____
7. Demonstrate sensitivity to the patient by showing empathy and clarifying that you understand what the patient is stating. Give the patient your full attention during the conversation and reserve judgment.	15	_____	_____	_____
8. Demonstrate sensitivity to the patient by using a pleasant, courteous tone of voice. Use body language to communicate respect (e.g., eye contact if culturally appropriate, keep arms uncrossed and relaxed).	15	_____	_____	_____
9. Provide the patient with options if appropriate.	10	_____	_____	_____

Comments:

Points earned _____ + 100 possible points = Score _____ % Score

Instructor's signature _____

PROCEDURE 17-2. PERFORM PRECERTIFICATION WITH DOCUMENTATION

MAERB/CAAHEP COMPETENCIES: VIII.P.3.
ABHES COMPETENCIES: 8.c.2.

TASK: Obtain preauthorization from a patient's insurance carrier for requested services or procedures and complete the prior authorization paper form.

EQUIPMENT AND SUPPLIES:
- **Paper method:** Patient's health record, prior authorization (precertification) request form (or Work Product 17-1), copy of patient's health insurance ID card, a pen
- **Electronic method:** SimChart for the Medical Office (SCMO)

Standards: Complete the procedure and all critical steps in _____ minutes with a minimum score of 85% within three attempts.

Scoring: Divide the points earned by the total possible points. Failure to perform a critical step, indicated by an asterisk (*), results in an unsatisfactory overall score.

Time began _____ Time ended _____ Total minutes: _____

Steps	Possible Points	Attempt 1	Attempt 2	Attempt 3
1. **Paper method:** Gather the health record, precertification/prior authorization request form, copy of the health insurance ID card, and a pen. **Electronic method:** Access the Simulation Playground in SCMO.	10	_____	_____	_____
2. Using the health record, determine the service or procedure that requires precertification/preauthorization.	10	_____	_____	_____
3. **Paper method:** Complete the precertification/prior authorization request form using a pen. **Electronic method:** Click on the Form Repository icon in SCMO. Select the Prior Authorization Request from the left Info Panel. Use the Patient Search button at the bottom to find the patient. Complete the remaining fields of the form.	60	_____	_____	_____
4. Proofread the completed form and make any necessary revisions.	10	_____	_____	_____
5. **Paper method:** File the document in the health record after it is faxed to the insurance carrier. **Electronic method:** Print and fax or electronically send the form to the insurance carrier and save the form to the patient's record.	10	_____	_____	_____

Comments:

Points earned _____ ÷ 100 possible points = Score _____ % Score

Instructor's signature _____

PROCEDURE 17-3 A. COMPLETE AN INSURANCE CLAIM FORM

MAERB/CAAHEP COMPETENCIES: VIII.P.4.
ABHES COMPETENCIES: 8.c.

TASK: To accurately complete a CMS-1500 Health Insurance Claim Form.

EQUIPMENT AND SUPPLIES:
- Patient's health record
- Copy of patient's insurance ID card or cards
- Patient registration/intake form
- Encounter form
- Insurance claims processing guidelines
- Blank CMS-1500 Health Insurance Claim Form (Work Product 17-2, 17-3, 17-4, 17-5)

Standards: Complete the procedure and all critical steps in _____ minutes with a minimum score of 85% within three attempts.

Scoring: Divide the points earned by the total possible points. Failure to perform a critical step, indicated by an asterisk (*), results in an unsatisfactory overall score.

Time began _____ **Time ended** _____ **Total minutes:** _____

Steps	Possible Points	Attempt 1	Attempt 2	Attempt 3
1. Gather the documents required to complete the claim form.	5	_____	_____	_____
2. Complete the claim form using a pen. Use capital letters. Do not use punctuation (commas or dollar signs) unless indicated in the insurance guidelines. Use a hyphen to hyphenate last names.	15	_____	_____	_____
3. Using the patient's health insurance ID card, determine the type of insurance and the insured's ID number. Enter this information into blocks 1 and 1a.	5	_____	_____	_____
4. Using the ID card, the encounter form, and the registration/intake form, determine the patient's information and insured's information. Accurately complete blocks 2, 3, 5, 6, 9, and 10 a–c by entering in the patient's information. Complete 4, 7, and 11 a–d with the insured's information.	10	_____	_____	_____
5. Complete blocks 12 and 13 by entering "signature on file" and the date.	5	_____	_____	_____
6. Accurately enter the physician or supplier information by completing blocks 14–23. Use the eight (8)-digit format (MM/DD/YYYY) when needed.	10	_____	_____	_____
7. Using the encounter form, complete block 24 and the appropriate blocks from 24A through 24H.	15	_____	_____	_____
8. Complete blocks 24I through 27 by entering information on the provider's or healthcare facility where the service was provided and the patient's account number. Check the correct box to indicate acceptance of assignment of benefits.	15	_____	_____	_____

Steps	Possible Points	Attempt 1	Attempt 2	Attempt 3
9. Complete blocks 28–29 by entering the total charges, total amount paid, and the total amount due. Complete blocks 31–33a by entering in the provider's and facility's information.	10	_____	_____	_____
10. Review the claim for accuracy and completeness before submitting. Correct any errors or missing information.	10	_____	_____	_____

Comments:

Points earned _____ ÷ 100 possible points = Score _____ % Score

Instructor's signature _____

PROCEDURE 17-3 B. COMPLETE AN ELECTRONIC INSURANCE CLAIM

MAERB/CAAHEP COMPETENCIES: VIII.P.4.
ABHES COMPETENCIES: 7.b., 8.c.

TASK: Accurately complete an electronic claim form.

EQUIPMENT AND SUPPLIES:
- Patient's health record
- Photocopy of patient's insurance ID card(s)
- Patient registration intake form
- Encounter form
- Claims processing guidelines
- SimChart for the Medical Office (SCMO)

Standards: Complete the procedure and all critical steps in _____ minutes with a minimum score of 85% within three attempts.

Scoring: Divide the points earned by the total possible points. Failure to perform a critical step, indicated by an asterisk (*), results in an unsatisfactory overall score.

Time began _____ Time ended _____ Total minutes: _____

Steps	Possible Points	Attempt 1	Attempt 2	Attempt 3
1. Access the Simulation Playground in SimChart for the Medical Office. On the Clinical Care tab, make an Office Visit. On the New Encounter screen, fill in today's date, select a visit type that is most appropriate to the scenario, and the provider indicated in the scenario. Click Save.	10	_____	_____	_____
2. Complete the Superbill.	20	_____	_____	_____

- In the Coding & Billing tab and on the Superbill (see left Info Panel), search for the patient. Verify the name and DOB. Select the patient and click on the Select button.

- Click on the Office Visit you created.

- Click on ICD-10 and then type in the ICD-10 code or use TruCode to find it.

- Rank the office visit and type in the fee.

- Add any remaining fees. Click on Save and Next as you move through the screens.

- Complete the insured and patient information and patient condition information.

- Click on the box before "I am ready to submit the Superbill." Click on Yes for signature on file and add in today's date.

- Click on the Save button. After you see the banner that it was saved, click on the Submit Superbill button. (Completing the ledger is optional for this procedure.)

Steps	Possible Points	Attempt 1	Attempt 2	Attempt 3
3. On the Coding & Billing tab, select Claim from the Info Panel. Search for the patient. Verify the name and DOB. Select the patient and click on the Select button. Click on the icon in the Action column next to the encounter that you just created.	5	_____	_____	_____
4. Review the autopopulated fields in the Patient Info, Provider Info, and Pay Info tabs. Enter any additional information required and click on Save before moving to the next tab.	10	_____	_____	_____
5. Click on the Encounter Notes tab. Review the autopopulated fields for accuracy.	15	_____	_____	_____

- For the HIPAA form on file, click on the Yes radio button and select the correct date.

- Document any other required information.

- Click on the Save button.

Steps	Possible Points	Attempt 1	Attempt 2	Attempt 3
6. Click on the Claim Info tab and review the autopopulated information.	10	_____	_____	_____

- Document any additional information.

- Click the Save button.

Steps	Possible Points	Attempt 1	Attempt 2	Attempt 3
7. Click on the Charge Capture tab.	15	_____	_____	_____

- Document the encounter date in the DOS From and DOS To columns.

- In the CPT/HCPCS field, enter the code or use TruCode to access the encoder.

- Document the place of service in the POS column. Click on Save.

- Document the diagnosis code (from the Encounter Notes tab) in the DX field and any modifiers in the M1, M2, and M3 columns. Add in the units and charges.

- Document any additional information.

Steps	Possible Points	Attempt 1	Attempt 2	Attempt 3
8. Proofread the claim. Revise any information needed.	10	_____	_____	_____
9. Click on the Submission tab. Click on the box by "I am ready to submit the Claim." Click on Yes by "Signature on file" and select the appropriate date. Click the Save button. Click the Submit Claim button.	5	_____	_____	_____

Comments:

Points earned _____ ÷ 100 possible points = **Score** _____ **% Score**

Instructor's signature _____

PROCEDURE 17-4. UTILIZE MEDICAL NECESSITY GUIDELINES: RESPOND TO A "MEDICAL NECESSITY DENIED" CLAIM

MAERB/CAAHEP COMPETENCIES: IX.P.3., VIII.P.4.
ABHES COMPETENCIES: 8.c.

TASK: Resolve the insurance company's denial of medical necessity.

EQUIPMENT AND SUPPLIES:
- **Paper method:** Patient's health record, copy of patient's insurance ID card or cards, patient registration/intake form, encounter form, blank CMS-1500 Health Insurance Claim Form (Work Product 17-6), and a pen
- **Electronic method:** SimChart for the Medical Office
- Insurance denial letter or scenario

Standards: Complete the procedure and all critical steps in _____ minutes with a minimum score of 85% within three attempts.

Scoring: Divide the points earned by the total possible points. Failure to perform a critical step, indicated by an asterisk (*), results in an unsatisfactory overall score.

Time began _____ **Time ended** _____ **Total minutes:** _____

Steps	Possible Points	Attempt 1	Attempt 2	Attempt 3
1. Review the insurance denial letter carefully. Compare the patient's information from the denial letter to the health record, claim, and encounter form. Look for errors in the patient's name and date of birth.	15	_____	_____	_____
2. Compare the insurance denial letter to the health record, claim, and encounter forms. Look for errors in the date of service, the diagnosis, and the procedure codes. The procedure must be medically necessary for the diagnosis indicated.	15	_____	_____	_____
3. Complete a claim (either CMS-1500 or an electronic claim) by entering in the information about the carrier, patient, and insured.	25	_____	_____	_____
4. Enter the information regarding the physician, procedures, and diagnosis. Make sure to include all of the information from the encounter.	25	_____	_____	_____
5. Proofread the claim form for accuracy before submitting the claim.	20	_____	_____	_____

Comments:

Points earned _____ ÷ 100 possible points = **Score** _____ **% Score**

Instructor's signature _____

PROCEDURE 17-5. INFORM A PATIENT OF FINANCIAL OBLIGATIONS FOR SERVICES RENDERED

MAERB/CAAHEP COMPETENCIES: VII.P.4., VII.A.1.
ABHES COMPETENCIES: 5.c., 8.c., 8.f.

TASK: Inform the patient of his/her financial obligation and demonstrate professionalism when discussing the patient's billing record.

EQUIPMENT AND SUPPLIES:
- Patient's account record
- Copy of patient's insurance card

Standards: Complete the procedure and all critical steps in _____ minutes with a minimum score of 85% within three attempts.

Scoring: Divide the points earned by the total possible points. Failure to perform a critical step, indicated by an asterisk (*), results in an unsatisfactory overall score.

Time began _____ Time ended _____ Total minutes: _____

Steps	Possible Points	Attempt 1	Attempt 2	Attempt 3
1. Determine the patient's financial responsibility under the insurance plan by reviewing the copy of the patient's insurance card.	10	_____	_____	_____
2. Determine the amount the patient owes by reviewing the patient's account record.	10	_____	_____	_____
3. Discuss the situation with the patient.	20	_____	_____	_____
4. Demonstrate professionalism when discussing the situation with the patient. Verbal and nonverbal communication should demonstrate patience, understanding, and sensitivity. The medical assistant should refrain from inappropriate and unprofessional behavior, including eye rolling, harsh words, disrespectful comments, and similar behaviors.	30	_____	_____	_____
5. Demonstrate professionalism by respectfully providing the patient with payment options based on the clinic's policies and what the patient can pay on a monthly basis.	30	_____	_____	_____

Comments:

Points earned _____ ÷ 100 possible points = **Score** _____ **% Score**

Instructor's signature _____

WORK PRODUCT 17-1. PRECERTIFICATION/PRIOR AUTHORIZATION FORM

To be used with Procedure 17-2.

Precertification / Prior Authorization Request form

Patient's Name:	Date of Birth:

Member ID number: _____

Insurance Carrier: _____

Insurance Fax Number: _____

Date: _____

Ordering Physician: _____

Clinic Name and Address: _____

Service Requested & Provider of Service Information:

Service Requested (describe):

Frequency of Service:

Starting Service Date: _____

Diagnosis: _____

Procedure: _____

Injury related? (Yes or No) _____

Date of Injury: _____

Provider of Service: _____

Agency Phone: _____

Agency Contact Name: _____

Medical Office Representative _____

Ending Service Date: _____

ICD-10 Code: _____

CPT Code(s): _____

Worker's Compensation related? (Yes or No) _____

Agency Name and Address of Service

Fax Number: _____

Completed and sent on: _____

For insurance carrier's use ONLY

Authorization Number: _____

Effective Date: _____ Expiration Date: _____

Name: _____ Date: _____

WORK PRODUCT 17-2. CMS-1500 HEALTH INSURANCE CLAIM FORM

To be used with Procedure 17-3 A

MAERB/CAAHEP COMPETENCIES: VIII.P.3.
ABHES COMPETENCIES: 8.c.2.

HEALTH INSURANCE CLAIM FORM

APPROVED BY NATIONAL UNIFORM CLAIM COMMITTEE (NUCC) 02/12

| | PICA | | | | | | | | PICA | |

1. MEDICARE (Medicare#) **MEDICAID** (Medicaid#) **TRICARE** (ID#/DoD#) **CHAMPVA** (Member ID#) **GROUP HEALTH PLAN** (ID#) **FECA BLK LUNG** (ID#) **OTHER** (ID#)   **1a. INSURED'S I.D. NUMBER** (For Program in Item 1)

2. PATIENT'S NAME (Last Name, First Name, Middle Initial)

3. PATIENT'S BIRTH DATE MM DD YY   **SEX** M ☐ F ☐

4. INSURED'S NAME (Last Name, First Name, Middle Initial)

5. PATIENT'S ADDRESS (No., Street)

6. PATIENT RELATIONSHIP TO INSURED Self ☐ Spouse ☐ Child ☐ Other ☐

7. INSURED'S ADDRESS (No., Street)

CITY   STATE

8. RESERVED FOR NUCC USE

CITY   STATE

ZIP CODE   TELEPHONE (Include Area Code) (   )

ZIP CODE   TELEPHONE (Include Area Code) (   )

9. OTHER INSURED'S NAME (Last Name, First Name, Middle Initial)

10. IS PATIENT'S CONDITION RELATED TO:

11. INSURED'S POLICY GROUP OR FECA NUMBER

a. OTHER INSURED'S POLICY OR GROUP NUMBER

a. EMPLOYMENT? (Current or Previous) ☐ YES ☐ NO

a. INSURED'S DATE OF BIRTH MM DD YY   SEX M ☐ F ☐

b. RESERVED FOR NUCC USE

b. AUTO ACCIDENT? ☐ YES ☐ NO   PLACE (State)

b. OTHER CLAIM ID (Designated by NUCC)

c. RESERVED FOR NUCC USE

c. OTHER ACCIDENT? ☐ YES ☐ NO

c. INSURANCE PLAN NAME OR PROGRAM NAME

d. INSURANCE PLAN NAME OR PROGRAM NAME

10d. CLAIM CODES (Designated by NUCC)

d. IS THERE ANOTHER HEALTH BENEFIT PLAN? ☐ YES ☐ NO   If yes, complete items 9, 9a, and 9d.

READ BACK OF FORM BEFORE COMPLETING & SIGNING THIS FORM.
12. PATIENT'S OR AUTHORIZED PERSON'S SIGNATURE I authorize the release of any medical or other information necessary to process this claim. I also request payment of government benefits either to myself or to the party who accepts assignment below.

SIGNED _____   DATE _____

13. INSURED'S OR AUTHORIZED PERSON'S SIGNATURE I authorize payment of medical benefits to the undersigned physician or supplier for services described below.

SIGNED _____

14. DATE OF CURRENT ILLNESS, INJURY, or PREGNANCY (LMP) MM DD YY   QUAL.

15. OTHER DATE QUAL.   MM DD YY

16. DATES PATIENT UNABLE TO WORK IN CURRENT OCCUPATION MM DD YY   FROM   TO   MM DD YY

17. NAME OF REFERRING PROVIDER OR OTHER SOURCE   17a.   17b. NPI

18. HOSPITALIZATION DATES RELATED TO CURRENT SERVICES MM DD YY   FROM   TO   MM DD YY

19. ADDITIONAL CLAIM INFORMATION (Designated by NUCC)

20. OUTSIDE LAB? ☐ YES ☐ NO $ CHARGES

21. DIAGNOSIS OR NATURE OF ILLNESS OR INJURY Relate A-L to service line below (24E)   ICD Ind.
A. _____ B. _____ C. _____ D. _____
E. _____ F. _____ G. _____ H. _____
I. _____ J. _____ K. _____ L. _____

22. RESUBMISSION CODE   ORIGINAL REF. NO.

23. PRIOR AUTHORIZATION NUMBER

24. A. DATE(S) OF SERVICE From / To MM DD YY MM DD YY	B. PLACE OF SERVICE	C. EMG	D. PROCEDURES, SERVICES, OR SUPPLIES (Explain Unusual Circumstances) CPT/HCPCS MODIFIER	E. DIAGNOSIS POINTER	F. $ CHARGES	G. DAYS OR UNITS	H. EPSDT Family Plan	I. ID. QUAL.	J. RENDERING PROVIDER ID. #
1								NPI	
2								NPI	
3								NPI	
4								NPI	
5								NPI	
6								NPI	

25. FEDERAL TAX I.D. NUMBER ☐ SSN ☐ EIN

26. PATIENT'S ACCOUNT NO.

27. ACCEPT ASSIGNMENT? (For govt. claims, see back) ☐ YES ☐ NO

28. TOTAL CHARGE $

29. AMOUNT PAID $

30. Rsvd for NUCC Use

31. SIGNATURE OF PHYSICIAN OR SUPPLIER INCLUDING DEGREES OR CREDENTIALS (I certify that the statements on the reverse apply to this bill and are made a part thereof.)

SIGNED   DATE

32. SERVICE FACILITY LOCATION INFORMATION
a. NPI   b.

33. BILLING PROVIDER INFO & PH # (   )
a. NPI   b.

NUCC Instruction Manual available at: www.nucc.org   **PLEASE PRINT OR TYPE**   APPROVED OMB-0938-1197 FORM 1500 (02-12)

Name: _____ Date: _____

WORK PRODUCT 17-3. CMS-1500 HEALTH INSURANCE CLAIM FORM

To be used with Procedure 17-3 A

MAERB/CAAHEP COMPETENCIES: VIII.P.4.
ABHES COMPETENCIES: 8.c.

HEALTH INSURANCE CLAIM FORM

APPROVED BY NATIONAL UNIFORM CLAIM COMMITTEE (NUCC) 02/12

◄ CARRIER ►

| | PICA | | | | | | | | PICA | |

1. MEDICARE (Medicare#) MEDICAID (Medicaid#) TRICARE (ID#/DoD#) CHAMPVA (Member ID#) GROUP HEALTH PLAN (ID#) FECA BLK LUNG (ID#) OTHER (ID#)   1a. INSURED'S I.D. NUMBER (For Program in Item 1)

2. PATIENT'S NAME (Last Name, First Name, Middle Initial)

3. PATIENT'S BIRTH DATE MM DD YY SEX M F

4. INSURED'S NAME (Last Name, First Name, Middle Initial)

5. PATIENT'S ADDRESS (No., Street)

6. PATIENT RELATIONSHIP TO INSURED Self Spouse Child Other

7. INSURED'S ADDRESS (No., Street)

CITY STATE

8. RESERVED FOR NUCC USE

CITY STATE

ZIP CODE TELEPHONE (Include Area Code) ( )

ZIP CODE TELEPHONE (Include Area Code) ( )

9. OTHER INSURED'S NAME (Last Name, First Name, Middle Initial)

10. IS PATIENT'S CONDITION RELATED TO:

11. INSURED'S POLICY GROUP OR FECA NUMBER

a. OTHER INSURED'S POLICY OR GROUP NUMBER

a. EMPLOYMENT? (Current or Previous) YES NO

a. INSURED'S DATE OF BIRTH MM DD YY SEX M F

b. RESERVED FOR NUCC USE

b. AUTO ACCIDENT? PLACE (State) YES NO

b. OTHER CLAIM ID (Designated by NUCC)

c. RESERVED FOR NUCC USE

c. OTHER ACCIDENT? YES NO

c. INSURANCE PLAN NAME OR PROGRAM NAME

d. INSURANCE PLAN NAME OR PROGRAM NAME

10d. CLAIM CODES (Designated by NUCC)

d. IS THERE ANOTHER HEALTH BENEFIT PLAN? YES NO If yes, complete items 9, 9a, and 9d.

READ BACK OF FORM BEFORE COMPLETING & SIGNING THIS FORM.
12. PATIENT'S OR AUTHORIZED PERSON'S SIGNATURE I authorize the release of any medical or other information necessary to process this claim. I also request payment of government benefits either to myself or to the party who accepts assignment below.

SIGNED _____ DATE _____

13. INSURED'S OR AUTHORIZED PERSON'S SIGNATURE I authorize payment of medical benefits to the undersigned physician or supplier for services described below.

SIGNED _____

14. DATE OF CURRENT ILLNESS, INJURY, or PREGNANCY (LMP) MM DD YY QUAL.

15. OTHER DATE QUAL. MM DD YY

16. DATES PATIENT UNABLE TO WORK IN CURRENT OCCUPATION MM DD YY FROM TO MM DD YY

17. NAME OF REFERRING PROVIDER OR OTHER SOURCE

17a. 17b. NPI

18. HOSPITALIZATION DATES RELATED TO CURRENT SERVICES MM DD YY FROM TO MM DD YY

19. ADDITIONAL CLAIM INFORMATION (Designated by NUCC)

20. OUTSIDE LAB? YES NO $ CHARGES

21. DIAGNOSIS OR NATURE OF ILLNESS OR INJURY Relate A-L to service line below (24E) ICD Ind.

A. ____ B. ____ C. ____ D. ____
E. ____ F. ____ G. ____ H. ____
I. ____ J. ____ K. ____ L. ____

22. RESUBMISSION CODE ORIGINAL REF. NO.

23. PRIOR AUTHORIZATION NUMBER

| 24. A. DATE(S) OF SERVICE | | | | | | B. PLACE OF SERVICE | C. EMG | D. PROCEDURES, SERVICES, OR SUPPLIES (Explain Unusual Circumstances) CPT/HCPCS MODIFIER | | E. DIAGNOSIS POINTER | F. $ CHARGES | G. DAYS OR UNITS | H. EPSDT Family Plan | I. ID. QUAL. | J. RENDERING PROVIDER ID. # |
From MM DD YY			To MM DD YY												
1														NPI	
2														NPI	
3														NPI	
4														NPI	
5														NPI	
6														NPI	

25. FEDERAL TAX I.D. NUMBER SSN EIN

26. PATIENT'S ACCOUNT NO.

27. ACCEPT ASSIGNMENT? (For govt. claims, see back) YES NO

28. TOTAL CHARGE $

29. AMOUNT PAID $

30. Rsvd for NUCC Use

31. SIGNATURE OF PHYSICIAN OR SUPPLIER INCLUDING DEGREES OR CREDENTIALS (I certify that the statements on the reverse apply to this bill and are made a part thereof.)

SIGNED _____ DATE _____

32. SERVICE FACILITY LOCATION INFORMATION

a. NPI b.

33. BILLING PROVIDER INFO & PH # ( )

a. NPI b.

◄ PATIENT AND INSURED INFORMATION ► ◄ PHYSICIAN OR SUPPLIER INFORMATION ►

NUCC Instruction Manual available at: www.nucc.org **PLEASE PRINT OR TYPE** APPROVED OMB-0938-1197 FORM 1500 (02-12)

Name: _____   Date: _____

WORK PRODUCT 17-4. CMS-1500 HEALTH INSURANCE CLAIM FORM

To be used with Procedure 17-3 A

MAERB/CAAHEP COMPETENCIES: IX.P.3., VIII.P.4.
ABHES COMPETENCIES: 8.c.

HEALTH INSURANCE CLAIM FORM

APPROVED BY NATIONAL UNIFORM CLAIM COMMITTEE (NUCC) 02/12

☐☐☐ PICA   PICA ☐☐☐

| 1. MEDICARE ☐ (Medicare#) | MEDICAID ☐ (Medicaid#) | TRICARE ☐ (ID#/DoD#) | CHAMPVA ☐ (Member ID#) | GROUP HEALTH PLAN ☐ (ID#) | FECA BLK LUNG ☐ (ID#) | OTHER ☐ (ID#) | 1a. INSURED'S I.D. NUMBER (For Program in Item 1) |

2. PATIENT'S NAME (Last Name, First Name, Middle Initial)

3. PATIENT'S BIRTH DATE MM | DD | YY   SEX M ☐ F ☐

4. INSURED'S NAME (Last Name, First Name, Middle Initial)

5. PATIENT'S ADDRESS (No., Street)

6. PATIENT RELATIONSHIP TO INSURED Self ☐ Spouse ☐ Child ☐ Other ☐

7. INSURED'S ADDRESS (No., Street)

CITY   STATE

8. RESERVED FOR NUCC USE

CITY   STATE

ZIP CODE   TELEPHONE (Include Area Code) ( )

ZIP CODE   TELEPHONE (Include Area Code) ( )

9. OTHER INSURED'S NAME (Last Name, First Name, Middle Initial)

10. IS PATIENT'S CONDITION RELATED TO:

11. INSURED'S POLICY GROUP OR FECA NUMBER

a. OTHER INSURED'S POLICY OR GROUP NUMBER

a. EMPLOYMENT? (Current or Previous) YES ☐ NO ☐

a. INSURED'S DATE OF BIRTH MM | DD | YY   SEX M ☐ F ☐

b. RESERVED FOR NUCC USE

b. AUTO ACCIDENT? YES ☐ NO ☐ PLACE (State)

b. OTHER CLAIM ID (Designated by NUCC)

c. RESERVED FOR NUCC USE

c. OTHER ACCIDENT? YES ☐ NO ☐

c. INSURANCE PLAN NAME OR PROGRAM NAME

d. INSURANCE PLAN NAME OR PROGRAM NAME

10d. CLAIM CODES (Designated by NUCC)

d. IS THERE ANOTHER HEALTH BENEFIT PLAN? YES ☐ NO ☐ If yes, complete items 9, 9a, and 9d.

READ BACK OF FORM BEFORE COMPLETING & SIGNING THIS FORM.

12. PATIENT'S OR AUTHORIZED PERSON'S SIGNATURE I authorize the release of any medical or other information necessary to process this claim. I also request payment of government benefits either to myself or to the party who accepts assignment below.

SIGNED _____   DATE _____

13. INSURED'S OR AUTHORIZED PERSON'S SIGNATURE I authorize payment of medical benefits to the undersigned physician or supplier for services described below.

SIGNED _____

14. DATE OF CURRENT ILLNESS, INJURY, or PREGNANCY (LMP) MM | DD | YY   QUAL.

15. OTHER DATE QUAL. MM | DD | YY

16. DATES PATIENT UNABLE TO WORK IN CURRENT OCCUPATION FROM MM | DD | YY TO MM | DD | YY

17. NAME OF REFERRING PROVIDER OR OTHER SOURCE

17a.
17b. NPI

18. HOSPITALIZATION DATES RELATED TO CURRENT SERVICES FROM MM | DD | YY TO MM | DD | YY

19. ADDITIONAL CLAIM INFORMATION (Designated by NUCC)

20. OUTSIDE LAB? YES ☐ NO ☐ $ CHARGES

21. DIAGNOSIS OR NATURE OF ILLNESS OR INJURY Relate A-L to service line below (24E)   ICD Ind.

A. |_____ B. |_____ C. |_____ D. |_____
E. |_____ F. |_____ G. |_____ H. |_____
I. |_____ J. |_____ K. |_____ L. |_____

22. RESUBMISSION CODE   ORIGINAL REF. NO.

23. PRIOR AUTHORIZATION NUMBER

24. A. DATE(S) OF SERVICE From MM DD YY To MM DD YY	B. PLACE OF SERVICE	C. EMG	D. PROCEDURES, SERVICES, OR SUPPLIES (Explain Unusual Circumstances) CPT/HCPCS MODIFIER	E. DIAGNOSIS POINTER	F. $ CHARGES	G. DAYS OR UNITS	H. EPSDT Family Plan	I. ID. QUAL.	J. RENDERING PROVIDER ID. #
1								NPI	
2								NPI	
3								NPI	
4								NPI	
5								NPI	
6								NPI	

25. FEDERAL TAX I.D. NUMBER   SSN ☐ EIN ☐

26. PATIENT'S ACCOUNT NO.

27. ACCEPT ASSIGNMENT? (For govt. claims, see back) YES ☐ NO ☐

28. TOTAL CHARGE $

29. AMOUNT PAID $

30. Rsvd for NUCC Use

31. SIGNATURE OF PHYSICIAN OR SUPPLIER INCLUDING DEGREES OR CREDENTIALS (I certify that the statements on the reverse apply to this bill and are made a part thereof.)

SIGNED _____   DATE _____

32. SERVICE FACILITY LOCATION INFORMATION

a.   b.

33. BILLING PROVIDER INFO & PH # ( )

a.   b.

NUCC Instruction Manual available at: www.nucc.org   *PLEASE PRINT OR TYPE*   APPROVED OMB-0938-1197 FORM 1500 (02-12)

WORK PRODUCT 17-5. CMS-1500 HEALTH INSURANCE CLAIM FORM

To be used with Procedure 17-3 A

HEALTH INSURANCE CLAIM FORM

APPROVED BY NATIONAL UNIFORM CLAIM COMMITTEE (NUCC) 02/12

CARRIER

| | PICA | | | | | | | | PICA | |

1. MEDICARE (Medicare#) MEDICAID (Medicaid#) TRICARE (ID#/DoD#) CHAMPVA (Member ID#) GROUP HEALTH PLAN (ID#) FECA BLK LUNG (ID#) OTHER (ID#)

1a. INSURED'S I.D. NUMBER (For Program in Item 1)

2. PATIENT'S NAME (Last Name, First Name, Middle Initial)

3. PATIENT'S BIRTH DATE MM DD YY SEX M F

4. INSURED'S NAME (Last Name, First Name, Middle Initial)

5. PATIENT'S ADDRESS (No., Street)

6. PATIENT RELATIONSHIP TO INSURED Self Spouse Child Other

7. INSURED'S ADDRESS (No., Street)

CITY STATE

8. RESERVED FOR NUCC USE

CITY STATE

ZIP CODE TELEPHONE (Include Area Code) ( )

ZIP CODE TELEPHONE (Include Area Code) ( )

9. OTHER INSURED'S NAME (Last Name, First Name, Middle Initial)

10. IS PATIENT'S CONDITION RELATED TO:

11. INSURED'S POLICY GROUP OR FECA NUMBER

a. OTHER INSURED'S POLICY OR GROUP NUMBER

a. EMPLOYMENT? (Current or Previous) YES NO

a. INSURED'S DATE OF BIRTH MM DD YY SEX M F

b. RESERVED FOR NUCC USE

b. AUTO ACCIDENT? PLACE (State) YES NO

b. OTHER CLAIM ID (Designated by NUCC)

c. RESERVED FOR NUCC USE

c. OTHER ACCIDENT? YES NO

c. INSURANCE PLAN NAME OR PROGRAM NAME

d. INSURANCE PLAN NAME OR PROGRAM NAME

10d. CLAIM CODES (Designated by NUCC)

d. IS THERE ANOTHER HEALTH BENEFIT PLAN? YES NO *If yes, complete items 9, 9a, and 9d.*

READ BACK OF FORM BEFORE COMPLETING & SIGNING THIS FORM.

12. PATIENT'S OR AUTHORIZED PERSON'S SIGNATURE I authorize the release of any medical or other information necessary to process this claim. I also request payment of government benefits either to myself or to the party who accepts assignment below.

SIGNED _____ DATE _____

13. INSURED'S OR AUTHORIZED PERSON'S SIGNATURE I authorize payment of medical benefits to the undersigned physician or supplier for services described below.

SIGNED _____

PATIENT AND INSURED INFORMATION

14. DATE OF CURRENT ILLNESS, INJURY, or PREGNANCY (LMP) MM DD YY QUAL.

15. OTHER DATE QUAL. MM DD YY

16. DATES PATIENT UNABLE TO WORK IN CURRENT OCCUPATION MM DD YY FROM TO MM DD YY

17. NAME OF REFERRING PROVIDER OR OTHER SOURCE 17a. 17b. NPI

18. HOSPITALIZATION DATES RELATED TO CURRENT SERVICES MM DD YY FROM TO MM DD YY

19. ADDITIONAL CLAIM INFORMATION (Designated by NUCC)

20. OUTSIDE LAB? YES NO $ CHARGES

21. DIAGNOSIS OR NATURE OF ILLNESS OR INJURY Relate A-L to service line below (24E) ICD Ind.

A. ____ B. ____ C. ____ D. ____
E. ____ F. ____ G. ____ H. ____
I. ____ J. ____ K. ____ L. ____

22. RESUBMISSION CODE ORIGINAL REF. NO.

23. PRIOR AUTHORIZATION NUMBER

24. A. DATE(S) OF SERVICE From MM DD YY To MM DD YY	B. PLACE OF SERVICE	C. EMG	D. PROCEDURES, SERVICES, OR SUPPLIES (Explain Unusual Circumstances) CPT/HCPCS MODIFIER	E. DIAGNOSIS POINTER	F. $ CHARGES	G. DAYS OR UNITS	H. EPSDT Family Plan	I. ID. QUAL.	J. RENDERING PROVIDER ID. #
1									NPI
2									NPI
3									NPI
4									NPI
5									NPI
6									NPI

25. FEDERAL TAX I.D. NUMBER SSN EIN

26. PATIENT'S ACCOUNT NO.

27. ACCEPT ASSIGNMENT? (For govt. claims, see back) YES NO

28. TOTAL CHARGE $

29. AMOUNT PAID $

30. Rsvd for NUCC Use

31. SIGNATURE OF PHYSICIAN OR SUPPLIER INCLUDING DEGREES OR CREDENTIALS (I certify that the statements on the reverse apply to this bill and are made a part thereof.)

SIGNED _____ DATE _____

32. SERVICE FACILITY LOCATION INFORMATION

a. NPI b.

33. BILLING PROVIDER INFO & PH # ( )

a. NPI b.

PHYSICIAN OR SUPPLIER INFORMATION

NUCC Instruction Manual available at: www.nucc.org

PLEASE PRINT OR TYPE

APPROVED OMB-0938-1197 FORM 1500 (02-12)

265

WORK PRODUCT 17-6. CMS-1500 HEALTH INSURANCE CLAIM FORM

To be used with Procedure 17-4.

HEALTH INSURANCE CLAIM FORM

APPROVED BY NATIONAL UNIFORM CLAIM COMMITTEE (NUCC) 02/12

| | PICA | | | | | | | | PICA | |

1. MEDICARE	MEDICAID	TRICARE	CHAMPVA	GROUP HEALTH PLAN	FECA BLK LUNG	OTHER	1a. INSURED'S I.D. NUMBER	(For Program in Item 1)
(Medicare#)	(Medicaid#)	(ID#/DoD#)	(Member ID#)	(ID#)	(ID#)	(ID#)		

2. PATIENT'S NAME (Last Name, First Name, Middle Initial)

3. PATIENT'S BIRTH DATE MM DD YY SEX M F

4. INSURED'S NAME (Last Name, First Name, Middle Initial)

5. PATIENT'S ADDRESS (No., Street)

6. PATIENT RELATIONSHIP TO INSURED Self Spouse Child Other

7. INSURED'S ADDRESS (No., Street)

CITY STATE

8. RESERVED FOR NUCC USE

CITY STATE

ZIP CODE TELEPHONE (Include Area Code) ( )

ZIP CODE TELEPHONE (Include Area Code) ( )

9. OTHER INSURED'S NAME (Last Name, First Name, Middle Initial)

10. IS PATIENT'S CONDITION RELATED TO:

11. INSURED'S POLICY GROUP OR FECA NUMBER

a. OTHER INSURED'S POLICY OR GROUP NUMBER

a. EMPLOYMENT? (Current or Previous) YES NO

a. INSURED'S DATE OF BIRTH MM DD YY SEX M F

b. RESERVED FOR NUCC USE

b. AUTO ACCIDENT? PLACE (State) YES NO

b. OTHER CLAIM ID (Designated by NUCC)

c. RESERVED FOR NUCC USE

c. OTHER ACCIDENT? YES NO

c. INSURANCE PLAN NAME OR PROGRAM NAME

d. INSURANCE PLAN NAME OR PROGRAM NAME

10d. CLAIM CODES (Designated by NUCC)

d. IS THERE ANOTHER HEALTH BENEFIT PLAN? YES NO If yes, complete items 9, 9a, and 9d.

READ BACK OF FORM BEFORE COMPLETING & SIGNING THIS FORM.
12. PATIENT'S OR AUTHORIZED PERSON'S SIGNATURE I authorize the release of any medical or other information necessary to process this claim. I also request payment of government benefits either to myself or to the party who accepts assignment below.

SIGNED _____ DATE _____

13. INSURED'S OR AUTHORIZED PERSON'S SIGNATURE I authorize payment of medical benefits to the undersigned physician or supplier for services described below.

SIGNED _____

14. DATE OF CURRENT ILLNESS, INJURY, or PREGNANCY (LMP) MM DD YY QUAL.

15. OTHER DATE QUAL. MM DD YY

16. DATES PATIENT UNABLE TO WORK IN CURRENT OCCUPATION MM DD YY FROM TO MM DD YY

17. NAME OF REFERRING PROVIDER OR OTHER SOURCE

17a. 17b. NPI

18. HOSPITALIZATION DATES RELATED TO CURRENT SERVICES MM DD YY FROM TO MM DD YY

19. ADDITIONAL CLAIM INFORMATION (Designated by NUCC)

20. OUTSIDE LAB? YES NO $ CHARGES

21. DIAGNOSIS OR NATURE OF ILLNESS OR INJURY Relate A-L to service line below (24E) ICD Ind.

A. ____ B. ____ C. ____ D. ____
E. ____ F. ____ G. ____ H. ____
I. ____ J. ____ K. ____ L. ____

22. RESUBMISSION CODE ORIGINAL REF. NO.

23. PRIOR AUTHORIZATION NUMBER

24. A. DATE(S) OF SERVICE		B. PLACE OF SERVICE	C. EMG	D. PROCEDURES, SERVICES, OR SUPPLIES (Explain Unusual Circumstances)		E. DIAGNOSIS POINTER	F. $ CHARGES	G. DAYS OR UNITS	H. EPSDT Family Plan	I. ID. QUAL.	J. RENDERING PROVIDER ID. #
From MM DD YY	To MM DD YY			CPT/HCPCS	MODIFIER						
1										NPI	
2										NPI	
3										NPI	
4										NPI	
5										NPI	
6										NPI	

25. FEDERAL TAX I.D. NUMBER SSN EIN

26. PATIENT'S ACCOUNT NO.

27. ACCEPT ASSIGNMENT? (For govt. claims, see back) YES NO

28. TOTAL CHARGE $

29. AMOUNT PAID $

30. Rsvd for NUCC Use

31. SIGNATURE OF PHYSICIAN OR SUPPLIER INCLUDING DEGREES OR CREDENTIALS (I certify that the statements on the reverse apply to this bill and are made a part thereof.)

SIGNED _____ DATE _____

32. SERVICE FACILITY LOCATION INFORMATION

a. NPI b.

33. BILLING PROVIDER INFO & PH # ( )

a. NPI b.

NUCC Instruction Manual available at: www.nucc.org

PLEASE PRINT OR TYPE

APPROVED OMB-0938-1197 FORM 1500 (02-12)

267

18 Patient Accounts, Collections, and Practice Management

VOCABULARY REVIEW

Fill in the blanks with the correct vocabulary terms from this chapter.

1. Dr. Martin is reviewing his _____, which lists the amounts charged by the provider for services rendered.

2. The Peete family was considered _____ _____, because they could not afford medical care even though they were able to pay basic living expenses.

3. Julie works with _____ _____, which is the money that is owed to the physicians.

4. Brigitte works with _____ _____, which is debt that has been incurred or owed by the provider to others.

5. _____ _____ _____ is used as a last resort option to collect payment from patients.

6. When a patient files for bankruptcy under Chapter 13, he or she will be paying a fixed dollar amount to a(n) _____ who will then pass the payment on to the creditors.

7. A(n) _____ will make financial decisions about the estate of a deceased patient.

8. A(n) _____ is the person who accepts financial responsibility for the patient.

9. Recording the charges a patient has incurred and the payments made on their account is _____.

10. When a provider's fee exceeds the allowed amount stated on the explanation of benefits from the insurance company a(n) _____ is posted to the patient account record for that difference.

11. When preparing to pay the monthly bills, Brigitte reviews the _____ from ABC Medical Supply Company, which lists the products that were provided to the medical office.

12. When using small claims court to collect a past due amount from a patient, Dr. Walden would be considered the _____.

13. When a patient writes a check to the medical office and does not have enough money in his or her checking account to cover it, the check will be returned to the medical office as _____ _____.

SKILLS AND CONCEPTS

1. What items should appear on the financial records of any business at all times?

   a. _____

   b. _____

   c. _____

   d. _____

269

2. Name two common accounting systems used in medical offices.

a. _____

b. _____

3. Examine the fee schedule and answer the following questions:

FEE SCHEDULE

BLACKBURN PRIMARY CARE ASSOCIATES, PC
1990 Turquiose Drive
Blackburn, WI 54937
608-459-8857

Federal Tax ID Number: 00-0000000   BCBS Group Number: 14982
                                             Medicare Group Number: 14982

OFFICE VISIT, NEW PATIENT

Focused, 99201	$45.00
Expanded, 99202	$55.00
Intermediate, 99203	$60.00
Extended, 99204	$95.00
Comprehensive, 99205	$195.00
Consultation, 99245	$250.00

OFFICE VISIT, ESTABLISHED PATIENT

Minimal, 99211	$40.00
Focused, 99212	$48.00
Intermediate, 99213	$55.00
Extended, 99214	$65.00
Comprehensive, 99215	$195.00

OFFICE PROCEDURES

EKG, 12 lead, 93000	$55.00
Stress EKG, Treadmill, 93015	$295.00
Sigmoidoscopy, Flex; 45330	$145.00
Spirometry, 94010	$50.00
Cerumen Removal, 69210	$40.00
Collection & Handling	
Lab Specimen, 99000	$9.00
Venipuncture, 35415	$9.00
Urinalysis, 81000	$20.00
Urinalysis, 81002 (Dip Only)	$12.00
Influenza Injection, 90724	$20.00
Pneumococcal Injection, 90732	$20.00
Oral Polio, 90712	$15.00
DTaP, 90700	$20.00
Tetanus Toxoid, 90703	$15.00
MMR, 90707	$25.00
HIB, 90737	$20.00
Hepatitis B, newborn to	
age 11 years, 90744	$60.00
Hepatitis B, 11-19 years, 90745	$60.00
Hepatitis B, 20 years and above	
90746	$60.00
Intramuscular Injection, 90788	
Penicillin	$30.00
Cephtriaxone	$25.00
Solu-Medrol	$23.00
Vitamin B-12	$13.00
Subcutaneous Injection, 90782	
Epinephrine	$18.00
Susphrine	$25.00
Insulin, U-100	$15.00

COMMON DIAGNOSTIC CODES

Ischemic Heart Disease	414.9
w/o myocardial infarction	411.89
w/coronary occlusion	411.81
Hypertension, Malignant	401.0
Benign	401.1
Unspecified	401.9
w/congest. heart failure	402.91
Asthma, Bronchial	493.9
w/COPD	493.2
allergic, w/S.A.	493.91
allergic, w/o S.A.	493.90
Kyphosis	737.10
w/osteoporosis	733.0
Osteoporosis	733.00
Otitis Media, Acute	382.9
Chronic	382.9

a. What is the charge for a consultation? _____

b. What is the charge for CPT code 99203? _____

c. What is the most expensive procedure on the list? _____

d. Which injection is more expensive, insulin or vitamin B_{12}? _____

4. What are the pitfalls of fee adjustments?

_____

_____

_____

5. What is professional courtesy and why is it less common now than in years past?

_____

_____

_____

6. Briefly explain how "skips" can be traced.

_____

_____

_____

7. Match the following terms with the correct definition:

Terms	Definitions
1. Accounts payable	A. Money that is expected but has not yet been received
2. Accounts receivable	B. Fees applied to the patient account when services are rendered
3. Adjustments	C. The management of debt incurred and not yet paid
4. Charges	D. Money given to the provider in exchange for services
5. Payments	E. Credits posted to the patient account when the provider's fee exceeds the amount allowed stated on the EOB

8. When a patient account is turned over to a collection agency, what adjustment is posted to the account?

_____

_____

_____

9. When a patient has a credit balance on his or her account, what adjustment is posted to the account?

_____

_____

_____

WORKPLACE APPLICATION

Complete this activity and share your results with the class, if appropriate.

Mr. Sanchez comes to the desk to check out after seeing the physician. When Brenda tells him that his bill is $95, he complains that he only saw the physician for 10 minutes. The fee is in accordance with evaluation and management guidelines. Explain the fees to Mr. Sanchez.

INTERNET ACTIVITIES

Complete one or more of these activities and share your results with the class, if appropriate.

1. Investigate bookkeeping software on the Internet and use any tutorials or trial software available. Determine a good program for use in the medical office and be able to defend your decision in a class presentation.

2. Research the role of an accountant and why most providers employ one to handle financials for the office. Discuss what the accountant does for the physician.

3. Investigate companies or banks that provide credit card financing for medical services in a physician's office. Talk about the types of offices that would most benefit from financing medical procedures.

4. Explore the fees that are often charged to the office for credit card transactions and discuss whether it is less expensive to process cards as debit cards or credit cards.

AFFECTIVE COMPETENCY: VII.A2. DISPLAY SENSITIVITY WHEN REQUESTING PAYMENT FOR SERVICES RENDERED

Explanation: Student must achieve a minimum score of 3 in each category to achieve competency.

Collecting money from patients can be a daunting task because many people are not comfortable talking about money, especially when they know that they have owed the provider for quite some time. It is important to display sensitivity to the situation when attempting to collect the money that is owed to the provider for services that have been rendered. Both your verbal and nonverbal communication must remain at a professional level, even if the patient's communication does not.

Using the following case study, role-play with a peer how you would display sensitivity when requesting payment for services rendered.

When reviewing the patients who are scheduled for appointments tomorrow you notice that Celia Tapia has an outstanding balance of $125 from charges that were incurred 5 months ago. It is office policy that patients with a balance owed for more than 120 days are not seen until the balance has been paid or payment arrangements have been made.

Scoring Criteria (1-4)	Excellent Evidence of Learning 4	Adequate Evidence of Learning 3	Limited Evidence of Learning 2	Unacceptable Evidence of Learning 1	Score Attempt 1	Score Attempt 2	Score Attempt 3
Demonstrated sensitive verbal communication by being respectful, honest, and showing courtesy	Student was respectful and courteous in his/her verbal communication while delivering a truthful sensitive message	Student was respectful and courteous in his/her verbal communication but the delivery of a truthful sensitive message needs improvement	Student awkwardly attempted to be respectful and courteous while delivering a truthful, sensitive message, but a lot more work is needed on the delivery and/or the tactful behaviors	Student's response was not respectful or courteous, thus the delivery of the message was unprofessional and lacked tact			
Displayed sensitive nonverbal behaviors when communicating with the patient	Student demonstrated nonverbal behaviors that reflect respect, compassion, diplomacy, and courtesy	Student demonstrated some nonverbal behaviors that reflect respect, compassion, diplomacy and courtesy, but a little more improvement is needed	Student demonstrated limited nonverbal behavior that reflected respect, compassion, diplomacy and courtesy, but a lot more improvement is needed	Student's nonverbal communication was perceived as being awkward, disrespectful, and/or unkind; lacking proper eye contact and/or normal tone of voice			

Comments:

AFFECTIVE COMPETENCY: VIII.A1. INTERACT PROFESSIONALLY WITH THIRD-PARTY REPRESENTATIVES

Explanation: Student must achieve a minimum score of 3 in each category to achieve competency.

It is often the responsibility of the medical assistant to interact with third-party representatives, such as the customer service representatives at an insurance company. You must maintain professional behaviors when dealing with all third-party representatives.

Using the following case study, role-play with a peer how you would interact professionally with third-party representatives.

Anna Richardson would like to schedule a tubal ligation, but is not sure if it is a covered benefit under her insurance policy. She would also like to know what her out-of-pocket expenses will be (how much of her deductible is left to be met, coinsurance, and copayment amounts).

Scoring Criteria (1-4)	Excellent Evidence of Learning 4	Adequate Evidence of Learning 3	Limited Evidence of Learning 2	Unacceptable Evidence of Learning 1	Score Attempt 1	Score Attempt 2	Score Attempt 3
Demonstrated sensitive verbal communication by being respectful, honest, and showing courtesy	Student was professional and courteous in his/her verbal communication	Student was professional and courteous in his/her verbal communication but the delivery of the message needs improvement	Student awkwardly attempted to be professional and courteous while delivering the message, but a lot more work is needed on the delivery and/or the tactful behaviors	Student's response was not professional or courteous, thus the delivery of the message was unprofessional and lacked tact			
Displayed sensitive nonverbal behaviors when communicating with the patient	Student demonstrated nonverbal behaviors that reflect professional communication	Student demonstrated some nonverbal behaviors that reflect professional communication, but a little more improvement is needed	Student demonstrated limited nonverbal behavior that reflected professional communication but a lot more improvement is needed	Student's nonverbal communication was perceived as being awkward, disrespectful, and/or unkind; tone of voice and/or other nonverbal behaviors			

Comments:

PROCEDURE 18-1. PERFORM ACCOUNTS RECEIVABLE PROCEDURES FOR PATIENT ACCOUNTS: CHARGES

MAERB/CAAHEP COMPETENCIES: VIII.P.1.
ABHES COMPETENCIES: 8.b.1.

TASK: Enter charges into the patient account record manually and electronically.

EQUIPMENT AND SUPPLIES:
- Patient account ledger card
- SimChart for the Medical Office software
- Encounter form/superbill
- Provider's fee schedule

Scenario 1: Ken Thomas is a returning patient of Dr. Martin. He is being seen for hypertension (ICD-10-CM; I10). He makes his $50 copayment at the time of the office visit.

Scenario 2: Martha Bravo is seeing Dr. Walden for the first time for hypothyroidism (ICD-10-CM; E03.9). She makes the $30 copayment at the time of the office visit.

Name:	Martha Bravo
Address:	1234 Anywhere Station Anywhere, Anystate 12345
Contact #1:	(212) 555-1212
Contact #2	(212) 555-1313
Emergency Contact:	John Bravo (212) 555-2627
SSN:	111-22-3333
DOB:	1/23/56
Health Insurance Information:	Carrier: Aetna Subscriber: Martha Bravo Subscriber DOB: 1/23/56 ID #: XEK3332328748 Group #: X1000 Effective Date: 1/1/20XX
Employer Information:	Name: Malibu Gardening Contact: (212) 555-5151

Standards: Complete the procedure and all critical steps in _____ minutes with a minimum score of 85% within three attempts.

Scoring: Divide the points earned by the total possible points. Failure to perform a critical step, indicated by an asterisk (*), results in an unsatisfactory overall score.

Time began _____ Time ended _____ Total minutes: _____

Steps	Possible Points	Attempt 1	Attempt 2	Attempt 3
1. For new patients, create the patient account by entering the following information on a patient account ledger card:	25	_____	_____	_____

- Patient's full name, address, and at least two contact phone numbers

- Date of birth

- Health insurance information, including the subscriber numbers, group number, and effective date

- Subscriber's name and date of birth (if the subscriber is not the patient)

- Employer's name and contact information

	Possible Points	Attempt 1	Attempt 2	Attempt 3
2. For returning patients, review the account record to see whether a balance is due. If there is a balance, bring this to the patient's attention when he or she comes for the appointment. Respectfully explain that the provider would appreciate a payment on the previous balance before he or she can care for the patient.	25	_____	_____	_____
Using the completed encounter form, enter the charges manually on the ledger card for the patient's account record.	50	_____	_____	_____

3. After seeing the patient, the provider completes the encounter form, which includes all procedures and the associated fee schedule.

Manual Method:

A. Total all the charges on the encounter form for the services rendered.

B. Then subtract the copayment made from the total charges. The previous balance, if any, is added to this new total.

Electronic Method Using SimChart:

A. After logging into SimChart, locate the established patient by clicking on Find Patient, enter the patient's name, verify DOB, and click on the radio button. This will bring you to the Clinical Care tab. If there is no encounter shown, create an encounter by clicking on Office Visit under Info Panel on the left, select a visit type and click on Save. Once an encounter has been created return to the Patient Dashboard and click on the Superbill link on the right (or click on the Coding and Billing tab).

B. From the Superbill area, in the Encounter Not Coded section, click on the encounter (in blue). On page 1 enter the diagnosis in the Diagnosis field and document the services provided (additional services are found on pages 2–3 of the superbill).

C. Complete the information needed on page 4 of the superbill and submit.

D. Click on Ledger on the left and search for your patient. Once your patient has been located click on the arrow across from the name in the ledger.

E. Enter the services provided and the payment received. Click on the Add Row button to continue to add services. The balance will be auto-calculated for you.

Comments:

Points earned _____ ÷ 100 possible points = Score _____ % Score

Instructor's signature _____

PROCEDURE 18-2. PERFORM ACCOUNTS RECEIVABLE PROCEDURES IN PATIENT ACCOUNTS: PAYMENTS AND ADJUSTMENTS

MAERB/CAAHEP COMPETENCIES: VIII.P.1.
ABHES COMPETENCIES: 8.b.1., 8.b.2.

TASK: Process payments and adjustments to patient account records accurately.

EQUIPMENT AND SUPPLIES
• Patient account ledger card or SimChart for the Medical Office software
• Explanation of benefits

Standards: Complete the procedure and all critical steps in _____ minutes with a minimum score of 85% within three attempts.

Scoring: Divide the points earned by the total possible points. Failure to perform a critical step, indicated by an asterisk (*), results in an unsatisfactory overall score.

Time began _____ **Time ended** _____ **Total minutes:** _____

Steps	Possible Points	Attempt 1	Attempt 2	Attempt 3
Posting Payments and Adjustments Manually	20	_____	_____	_____
1. Review the EOB for multiple patient accounts received by the healthcare facility.				
2. Look up the ledger card for the patient account (or the patient ledger in SimChart).	40	_____	_____	_____
3. Post the payment and adjustment line by line.	40	_____	_____	_____
Posting Payments and Adjustments in SimChart	20	_____	_____	_____
1. After one line on the EOB has been posted, post all subsequent lines on the EOB separately.				
2. Confirm that the adjustment was necessary on the EOB. Review the amount paid. If there is concern that the amount adjusted was too much, either review the provider's contract with the insurance company's fee schedule to compare payments, or call the insurance company's provider services to inquire about the applicable adjusted amount.	40	_____	_____	_____
3. When the patient's financial responsibility has been established, send the patient a statement. The secondary insurance should be billed if the patient is covered.	40	_____	_____	_____

Comments:

Points earned _____ ÷ 100 possible points = Score _____ % Score

Instructor's signature _____

Chapter **18** **Patient Accounts, Collections, and Practice Management**

Ledger:

Blue Cross Blue Shield					
ID # KT4496785					
Group # 55124T					
Subscriber: Ken Thomas		Ken Thomas			
		398 Larkin Avenue			
DOB: 10/25/1961		Anytown, Anystate 12345-1234			

Date	Service Description	Charges	Payments	Adjustments	Balance
06/03/20XX	99204	250.00			250.00
06/03/20XX	94375	40.00			290.00
06/03/20XX	94060	75.00			365.00
06/03/20XX	94664	50.00			415.00
06/03/20XX	94760	50.00			465.00

BLUE CROSS BLUE SHIELD
1234 Insurance Place
Anytown, Anystate 12345-1234

Claim Number:	1-99-16987087
Group Name:	ABC Company
Group Number:	55124T

Employee:	Ken Thomas
Patient:	Ken Thomas
SSN:	783212215
Prepared by:	M. Smith
Prepared on:	07/04/20xx

James Martin, M.D.
Walden-Martin Family Medical Clinic

1234 Anystreet
Anytown, Anystate 12345-1234

PATIENT RESPONSIBILITY

Amount not covered:	0.00
Co-pay amount:	0.00
Deductible:	0.00
Coinsurance:	64.61
Patient's total responsibility	64.61

EXPLANATION OF BENEFITS

DOS	CPT/HCPCS	Charge Amount	Not Covered	Reason Code	PPO Discount	Covered Amount	Ded Amount	Copay	Paid at	Payment Amount
06/03/20xx	99204	250.00	0.00	48	136.00	114.00	0.00	0.00	80%	91.20
06/03/20xx	94375	40.00	0.00	48	0.00	40.00	0.00	0.00	80%	32.00
06/03/20xx	94060	75.00	0.00	48	0.00	75.00	0.00	0.00	80%	60.00
06/03/20xx	94664	50.00	0.00	48	1.55	48.45	0.00	0.00	80%	38.76
06/03/20xx	94760	50.00	0.00	48	4.40	45.60	0.00	0.00	80%	36.48
TOTAL		465.00	0.00		141.95	323.05	0.00	0.00		258.44

Total Payment Amount   258.44

CPT Code

99204 OFFICE/OUTPT VISIT E/M NEW MOD-HI SEVERIT
94375 RESPIRATORY FLOW VOLUM LOOP
94060 BRONCHOSPSM EVAL SPIROM PRE and POST BRON
94664 AEROSOL/VAPOR FOR INHALA; INT DEMO and EVAL
94760 NONINVASIVE EAR/PULSE OXIMETRY-02 SAT

If you have any questions, call Blue Cross Blue Shield at (800) 255-9091

Reason Code

48 CON DISCOUNT/PT NOT RESPONSIBLE

19 Banking Services and Procedures

VOCABULARY REVIEW

Fill in the blanks with the correct vocabulary terms from the list.

1. A check that is not honored by the bank issuing the check because there were not sufficient funds in the entity's bank account or the account has been closed _____

2. The misuse of a healthcare facility's funds for personal gain _____ _____

3. A payment the bank makes in exchange for using money _____ _____

4. Money in a bank account that is not assigned to pay for any office expenses _____

5. A bank draft or an order to pay a certain sum of money on demand to a specified person or entity _____

6. Global technology that includes embedded microchips that store and protect cardholder data _____

7. A document used to withdraw money from one bank account and deposit it into another _____

8. The bank on which the check is drawn or written _____

9. A bank account against which checks can be written and funds can be transferred to the payable party _____

10. The person who signs his or her name on the back of a check for the purpose of transferring all rights in the check to another party _____

11. A capital sum of money due as a debt or used as a fund for which interest is either charged or paid _____

12. The person presenting the check for payment _____

13. Nine-digit code printed on the bottom left side of checks that identifies the bank upon which the check was drawn _____

a. Check
b. Checking account
c. Discretionary income
d. Drawee
e. Endorser
f. Embezzlement
g. EMV chip technology
h. Holder
i. Interest
j. Negotiable instruments
k. Nonsufficient funds check
l. Principal
m. Routing transit number

SKILLS AND CONCEPTS

Part I: Short Answers

1. Describe the following types of banking fees.

   a. Account maintenance fee:

   _____

   _____

b. Overdraft fee:

_____

_____

c. Nonsufficient funds fee:

_____

_____

d. Transaction fee:

_____

_____

2. In the ambulatory care setting, what is the checking account used for?

_____

_____

3. In the ambulatory care setting, what is a savings account used for?

_____

_____

4. You are a medical assistant in a small practice and have been told that you now have the responsibility for paying the bills by writing out and signing the checks. What is the first action you need to take before writing out the first check?

_____

_____

5. Name six activities that can be done with basic online banking services.

a. _____

b. _____

c. _____

d. _____

e. _____

f. _____

6. List the four requirements for a check to be negotiable.

a. _____

b. _____

c. _____

d. _____

7. Name five documents that can be used to withdraw money from one bank account and deposit it into another.

a. _____

b. _____

c. _____

d. _____

e. _____

8. Describe five precautions for accepting checks in the healthcare facility.

a. _____

b. _____

c. _____

d. _____

e. _____

9. Describe the adjustments that are made to the patient's account when an NSF check is received by the healthcare facility.

_____

_____

10. Describe four precautions to take if a patient is paying with cash.

a. _____

b. _____

c. _____

d. _____

11. Describe precautions to take when a patient pays with a debit card or a credit card.

_____

_____

_____

12. Describe the banking procedures as related to the ambulatory care setting and include the medical assistant's role with each procedure:

a. Making bank deposits:

_____

_____

b. Preparing a bank deposit:

_____

_____

c. Endorsing checks:

_____

_____

d. Writing checks:

_____

_____

e. Bank statement reconciliation:

_____

_____

13. Why is it important to make bank deposits of cash and checks daily?

_____

_____

_____

14. Describe three ways to do a mobile deposit of a check.

    a. _____

    b. _____

    c. _____

15. Describe each type of endorsement.

    a. Blank endorsement:

_____

_____

    b. Restrictive endorsement:

_____

_____

    c. Special endorsement:

_____

_____

16. With regard to checks, define stop-payment.

_____

_____

17. List three reasons a stop-payment would be done.

    a. _____

    b. _____

    c. _____

18. Define direct deposit.

_____

_____

19. If a mistake is made when preparing a check, what should be done?

_____

_____

20. What is a fidelity bond?

_____

_____

Part II: Preparing a Bank Deposit

Activity 1

Prepare a bank deposit ticket (slip) using Procedure 19-1 and Work Products 19-1 and 19-2. On the deposit ticket, write the following information: check and currency details, totals, and deposit date. Use the endorsement box on Work Product 19-2 to write a restrictive endorsement.

1. Checks to be deposited:
   - #2387 for $67 from Sue Patrick
   - #460 for $50 from Ronald Rodriguez
   - #3654 for $75 from Sam Brown
   - #598 for $25 from Debby Green
   - #695 for $35 from Dean Smith
   - #309 for $1203.30 for an insurance payment for Betty Perry
   - Total for checks: _____

2. Currency:
   - (22) $20 bills
   - (3) $50 bills
   - (68) $1 bills
   - (20) $10 bills
   - (46) $5 bills
   - Total for currency: _____

3. Coins:
   - (23) nickels
   - (52) quarters
   - (123) pennies
   - Total for coins: _____

4. Total deposited: _____

5. Practice writing a restrictive endorsement using the image on Work Product 19-2. Use the clinic name, bank name, and the account number found on Work Product 19-1.

Activity 2

Prepare a bank deposit ticket (slip) using Procedure 19-1 and Work Products 19-3 and 19-4. On the deposit ticket, write the following information: check and currency details, totals, and deposit date. Use the endorsement box on Work Product 19-4 to write a restrictive endorsement.

1. Checks to be deposited: #3456 for $89; #6954 for $136; #9854-10 for $1366.65; #8546 for $653.36; and #9865 for $890.22. Total for checks: _____

2. The following currency needs to be deposited: (19) $20 bills; (10) $10 bills; (46) $5 bills; (73) $1 bills. Total for currency: _____

3. Coins to be deposited: (43) quarters and (155) nickels. Total for coins: _____

4. Total deposited: _____

5. Practice writing a restrictive endorsement using the image on Work Product 19-4. Use the clinic name, bank name, and the account number found on Work Product 19-3.

Part III: Managing the Healthcare Facility Business Bank Account

For this activity, you will use Work Product 19-5—Checks. You will need to write out checks when indicated (use the checks on Work Product 19-5) and complete the log to the left side of the check image. Use today's date for the date. Keep a running balance as you complete the activity and fill in the running balances on the lines.

Beginning balance in checkbook is $5,302.66.

1. Write check #5648 to American Medical Supplies for $528.36 for supplies. Balance _____

2. Write check #5649 to Blackburn Utility Company for $66.89 to pay the water bill. Balance _____

3. Write check #5650 to Blackburn National Bank for $2,200 for the office rent payment. Balance _____

4. Write check #5651 to American Drug Supply for $1265.34 to pay a bill for medications. Balance _____

5. A deposit of third-party insurance checks of $2,358 was made. Balance _____

6. Credit card payments deposited were: $75, $100, and $250. Balance _____

Part IV: Reconciling a Bank Statement

Reconcile the bank statement using the following facts and figures. Use the worksheet in Work Product 19-6 to show your work.

The checkbook balance is $2,313.63. The statement balance is $3,324.79.

1. Three checks are outstanding: check #5648 for $426; check #5649 for $36.90; and check #5650 for $1,350. What is the total for outstanding checks? _____

2. Add in two deposits showing in the checkbook balance that do not show on the statement: $269.30 and $532.44. What is the total for deposits not listed? _____

3. Does the checkbook reconcile with the statement? _____

4. What is the ending balance on the worksheet? _____

CASE STUDY

The Internet has changed the way business is conducted both in the United States and beyond U.S. borders. Some individuals are quite comfortable making purchases and paying bills online. How safe are these practices? How can the medical assistant know that online bill-paying services are safe and secure? Research some online security features websites use to protect financial information online, and prepare a report.

INTERNET ACTIVITIES

Complete one or more of these activities and share your results with the class, if appropriate.

1. Research safety measures designed to keep confidential banking information private. How do privacy policies affect Internet banking? How can the medical assistant ensure that confidential information remains private? Prepare a paper or report for the class on this subject.

2. Explore mobile deposit technology and share your findings with the class.

3. What is the Federal Check 21 law? Determine how this legislation affects individuals and businesses. Share the information with the class.

PROCEDURE 19-1. PREPARE A BANK DEPOSIT

CAAHEP COMPETENCIES: VII.P.2.
ABHES COMPETENCIES: 8.b.

TASK: Prepare a bank deposit for checks, currency, and coins.

EQUIPMENT AND SUPPLIES:
- Checks, currency, and coins for deposit
- Check for endorsement (Work Products 19-2 and 19-4)
- Calculator
- **Paper method:** Bank deposit slip (Work Products 19-1 and 19-3)
- **Electronic method:** SimChart for the Medical Office (SCMO)

Standards: Complete the procedure and all critical steps in _____ minutes with a minimum score of 85% within three attempts.

Scoring: Divide the points earned by the total possible points. Failure to perform a critical step, indicated by an asterisk (*), results in an unsatisfactory overall score.

Time began _____ Time ended _____ Total minutes: _____

Steps	Possible Points	Attempt 1	Attempt 2	Attempt 3
1. Gather the documents to be used. For the paper method, use the paper bank deposit slip (Work Product 19-1 or 19-3). For the electronic method, enter into the Simulation Playground in SCMO. Click on the Form Repository icon. On the Info Panel, click on Office Forms and then select Bank Deposit Slip.	5	_____	_____	_____
2. Add the date on the deposit slip.	5	_____	_____	_____
3. Using the calculator, calculate the amount of currency to be deposited. Enter the amount in the Currency line, completing the dollar and cent boxes.	10	_____	_____	_____
4. Calculate the amount of coins to be deposited. Enter the amount in the Coin line, completing the dollar and cent boxes.	10	_____	_____	_____
5. Add the currency and coins and enter the total amount in the Total Cash line.	10	_____	_____	_____
6. For each check to be deposited, enter the check number, the dollars, and cents. List each check on a separate line.	20	_____	_____	_____
*7. Calculate the total to be deposited and enter the number in the Total From Attached List box.	10	_____	_____	_____
8. Enter the number of items deposited in the Total Items box.	10	_____	_____	_____
9. Verify the check amounts listed and recalculate the totals before completing the deposit slip. For the electronic method, click on Save.	10	_____	_____	_____
10. Place a restrictive endorsement on the check(s) (Work Product 19-2 or 19-4).	10	_____	_____	_____

Comments:

Points earned _____ ÷ 100 possible points = Score _____ % Score

Instructor's signature _____

Name: _____ Date: _____

WORK PRODUCT 19-1. BANK DEPOSIT SLIP

CAAHEP COMPETENCIES: VII.P.2.
ABHES COMPETENCIES: 8.b.

To be used with Procedure 19-1

Use this work product for Part II: Preparing a Bank Deposit, Activity 1.

DEPOSIT TICKET

WALDEN-MARTIN FAMLY MEDICAL CLINIC
1234 ANYSTREET
ANYTOWN, ANYSTATE 12345

DEPOSITS MAY NOT BE AVAILABLE FOR
IMMEDIATE WITHDRAWAL

Clear Water Bank
Anytown, Anystate

ACCOUNT NUMBER: 123-456-78910

Endorse & List Checks Separately

DATE _____	Dollars	Cents
CURRENCY		
COIN		
TOTAL CASH		
1.		
2.		
3.		
4.		
5.		
6.		
7.		
8.		
9.		
10.		
11.		
12.		
Less Cash Returned		
Total Items		Total Deposit	

WORK PRODUCT 19-2. ENDORSING A CHECK

CAAHEP COMPETENCIES: VII.P.2.
ABHES COMPETENCIES: 8.b.

To be used with Procedure 19-1

Use this work product for Part II: Preparing a Bank Deposit, Activity 1.

ENDORSE CHECK HERE

X

DO NOT WRITE STAMP, OR SIGN BELOW THIS LINE

WORK PRODUCT 19-3. PREPARE A BANK DEPOSIT

CAAHEP COMPETENCIES: VII.P.2.
ABHES COMPETENCIES: 8.b.

To be used with Procedure 19-1

Use this work product for Part II: Preparing a Bank Deposit, Activity 2.

DEPOSIT TICKET		
WALDEN-MARTIN FAMLY MEDICAL CLINIC **1234 ANYSTREET** **ANYTOWN, ANYSTATE 12345** DEPOSITS MAY NOT BE AVAILABLE FOR IMMEDIATE WITHDRAWAL Clear Water Bank Anytown, Anystate ACCOUNT NUMBER: 123-456-78910 Endorse & List Checks Separately		
DATE _____	Dollars	Cents
CURRENCY		
COIN		
TOTAL CASH		
1.		
2.		
3.		
4.		
5.		
6.		
7.		
8.		
9.		
10.		
11.		
12.		
Less Cash Returned		
Total Items	Total Deposit	

WORK PRODUCT 19-4. ENDORSING A CHECK

CAAHEP COMPETENCIES: VII.P.2.
ABHES COMPETENCIES: 8.b.

To be used with Procedure 19-1

Use this work product for Part II: Preparing a Bank Deposit, Activity 2.

ENDORSE CHECK HERE
X
DO NOT WRITE STAMP, OR SIGN BELOW THIS LINE

WORK PRODUCT 19-5. CHECKS

ABHES COMPETENCIES: 8.b.

Use this work product for Part III: Managing the Healthcare Facility Business Bank **Account**.

5648

DATE _____
TO _____
FOR _____

BALANCE BROUGHT FORWARD		
DEPOSITS		
BALANCE		
AMT THIS CK		
BALANCE CARRIED FORWARD		

BLACKBURN PRIMARY CARE ASSOCIATES, PC
1990 Turquoise Drive
Blackburn, WI 54937
608-459-8857

5648
94-72/1224

DATE _____

$ _____

PAY TO THE
ORDER OF _____

_____ DOLLARS

DERBYSHIRE SAVINGS
Member FDIC
P.O. BOX 8923
Blackburn, WI 54937

FOR _____

⑆055003⑆ 446782011⑆ 678800470

5649

DATE _____
TO _____
FOR _____

BALANCE BROUGHT FORWARD		
DEPOSITS		
BALANCE		
AMT THIS CK		
BALANCE CARRIED FORWARD		

BLACKBURN PRIMARY CARE ASSOCIATES, PC
1990 Turquoise Drive
Blackburn, WI 54937
608-459-8857

5649
94-72/1224

DATE _____

$ _____

PAY TO THE
ORDER OF _____

_____ DOLLARS

DERBYSHIRE SAVINGS
Member FDIC
P.O. BOX 8923
Blackburn, WI 54937

FOR _____

⑆055003⑆ 446782011⑆ 678800470

5650

DATE _____
TO _____
FOR _____

BALANCE BROUGHT FORWARD		
DEPOSITS		
BALANCE		
AMT THIS CK		
BALANCE CARRIED FORWARD		

BLACKBURN PRIMARY CARE ASSOCIATES, PC
1990 Turquoise Drive
Blackburn, WI 54937
608-459-8857

5650
94-72/1224

DATE _____

$ _____

PAY TO THE
ORDER OF _____

_____ DOLLARS

DERBYSHIRE SAVINGS
Member FDIC
P.O. BOX 8923
Blackburn, WI 54937

FOR _____

⑆055003⑆ 446782011⑆ 678800470

5651

DATE _____
TO _____
FOR _____

BALANCE BROUGHT FORWARD		
DEPOSITS		
BALANCE		
AMT THIS CK		
BALANCE CARRIED FORWARD		

BLACKBURN PRIMARY CARE ASSOCIATES, PC
1990 Turquoise Drive
Blackburn, WI 54937
608-459-8857

5651
94-72/1224

DATE _____

$ _____

PAY TO THE
ORDER OF _____

_____ DOLLARS

DERBYSHIRE SAVINGS
Member FDIC
P.O. BOX 8923
Blackburn, WI 54937

FOR _____

⑆055003⑆ 446782011⑆ 678800470

Name: _____ Date: _____

WORK PRODUCT 19-6. RECONCILING WORKSHEET

ABHES COMPETENCIES: 8.b.

Use this work product for Part IV: Reconciling a Bank Statement.

THIS WORKSHEET IS PROVIDED TO HELP YOU BALANCE YOUR ACCOUNT

1. Go through your register and mark each check, withdrawal, Express ATM transaction, payment, deposit, or other credit listed on this statement. Be sure that your register shows any interest paid into your account, and any service charges, automatic payments, or Express Transfers withdrawn from your account during this statement period.

2. Using the chart below, list any outstanding checks, Express ATM withdrawals, payments, or any other withdrawals (including any from previous months) that are listed in your register but are not shown on this statement.

3. Balance your account by filling in the spaces below.

ITEMS OUTSTANDING		
NUMBER	**AMOUNT**	
TOTAL	$	

ENTER

The NEW BALANCE shown on
this statement_____$

ADD

Any deposits listed in your register $
or transfers into your account $
which are not shown on this $
statement.   + $ _____

TOTAL

CALCULATE THE SUBTOTAL_____$

➤**SUBTRACT**

The total outstanding checks and
withdrawals from the chart at left_____-$

CALCULATE THE ENDING BALANCE

This amount should be the same
as the current balance shown in
your check register_____$

301

20 Supervision and Human Resources Management

VOCABULARY REVIEW

Fill in the blank with the correct vocabulary term from the list.

1. A term referring to actions taken by management to keep good employees.
   _____

2. Things that incite or spur to action; rewards or reasons for performing a task.
   _____

3. Ensuring that the healthcare facility meets standards and regulations according to the office's established policies and procedures. _____

4. A series of executive positions in order of authority. _____

5. Submissive to or controlled by authority; placed in or occupying a lower class, rank, or position. _____

6. Completely obvious, conspicuous, or obtrusive, especially in a crass or offensive manner; brazen. _____

7. Sticking together tightly; exhibiting or producing cohesion.
   _____

8. A student working in an ambulatory care environment who is learning the job and not earning a wage. _____

9. A steady employee whom a new staff member can approach with questions and concerns. _____

10. Slighting; having a negative or degrading tone. _____

11. Exhaustion of physical or emotional strength or motivation, usually as a result of prolonged stress or frustration. _____

12. Pleasant and at ease in talking to others; characterized by ease and friendliness.
    _____

13. The inclusion of every individual—regardless of age, religion, race, disability, and/or gender—in the medical practice. _____

14. Contains all documents related to an individual's employment.
    _____

15. To delegate more responsibilities to employees (a management theory).
    _____

a. Affable
b. Blatant
c. Burnout
d. Chain of command
e. Cohesive
f. Compliance
g. Disparaging
h. Diversity
i. Empower
j. Extern
k. Human resources file
l. Incentives
m. Mentor
n. Retention
o. Subordinate

SKILLS AND CONCEPTS

Part I: Short Answer Questions

1. List six qualities of an effective manager.

   a. _____

   b. _____

   c. _____

   d. _____

   e. _____

   f. _____

2. What is the advantage for a provider to hire a trustworthy, reliable, office manager to run the daily business aspects of the office?

   _____

   _____

3. Name six tasks that could be performed by the medical office manager.

   a. _____

   b. _____

   c. _____

   d. _____

   e. _____

   f. _____

4. When there is a chain of command in a healthcare facility, whom should the medical assistant go to first?

   _____

   _____

5. When there is a chain of command in a healthcare facility, to whom does the supervisor or office manager report?

   _____

6. List three incentives that would motivate you to do a good job in a position.

   a. _____

   b. _____

   c. _____

7. What occurs that improves communication in the healthcare workplace?

   _____

   _____

8. Name two positive things that occur when communication improves in the healthcare workplace.

   a. _____

   b. _____

9. Name two actions an office manager can take to improve employee morale.

a. _____

b. _____

10. Describe the following barriers to communication and explain how to overcome these barriers.

a. Physical separation barriers

_____

_____

_____

b. Language barriers

_____

_____

_____

c. Status barriers

_____

_____

_____

d. Gender difference barriers

_____

_____

_____

e. Cultural diversity barriers

_____

_____

_____

11. List five things that you can do to prevent burnout.

a. _____

b. _____

c. _____

d. _____

e. _____

12. List three effective methods for finding new employees.

a. _____

b. _____

c. _____

13. Explain the importance of giving all the interviewees the same questions during the interview.

_____

305

14. List five illegal interview questions.

a. _____

b. _____

c. _____

d. _____

e. _____

15. List five legal interview questions.

a. _____

b. _____

c. _____

d. _____

e. _____

16. Discuss topic areas that would be considered illegal and legal during an interview.

_____

_____

_____

17. Explain the importance of waiting until the job offer is accepted before informing applicants of the status of the position.

_____

_____

_____

Part II: Prepare for a Staff Meeting

For this activity, use Procedure 20-1 and the following scenario.

Scenario: You are a medical assistant team leader in a family practice department. Over the last two months there has been an increase in patient complaints related to long wait times in the reception area before being brought back to the patient exam rooms. Your supervisor asks you to prepare for a staff meeting to discuss these complaints and find ways to increase patient satisfaction.

CASE STUDY

You are a supervisor preparing to interview applicants for a front office scheduler position. Create 15 legal questions to ask the applicants. You should have straightforward questions, 2-3 (or more) behavioral questions and 2-3 (or more) situational questions.

WORK APPLICATIONS

Complete one or more of these activities and share your results with the class, if appropriate.

1. Create a job description or job posting for a "dream" job of your choice. Make sure to include the duties, required education, and other details typically found in postings.

2. Create a plan of how to screen applications and résumés for a medical assistant job in a family practice department. Describe the process you would use to evidentially identify the few applicants who should be interviewed.

Complete one or more of these activities and share your results with the class, if appropriate.

1. Research the I-9 form and summarize the process of completing the I-9 form.

2. Research the I-9 form and describe the acceptable forms used to complete the form.

3. Search the Internet for employment laws that pertain specifically to your state.

4. Select one employment law from this chapter and research it on the Internet. Look for real-life cases in which the law was breached, including any court action or rulings that pertain to the law. Share the information you find with the class.

5. Find team-building exercises designed to promote and build teamwork for a group of employees. Share the exercises with the class and select several of them to try with classmates. Briefly critique each one, determining how the exercise benefits the employees.

AFFECTIVE COMPETENCY: V.A.3.A–F. DEMONSTRATE RESPECT FOR INDIVIDUAL DIVERSITY, INCLUDING GENDER, RACE, RELIGION, AGE, ECONOMIC STATUS, AND APPEARANCE

Explanation: Student must achieve a minimum of a score of 3 in each category to achieve the related competency.

When working with patients who are different than you, it is important to treat them with respect and in the same manner you would want to be treated. Often if we are uncomfortable with the differences, it can be reflected in our verbal communication and nonverbal body language. Our patients can sense the tension and become uncomfortable and experience other negative feelings.

To demonstrate respect for all patients, it is important to do the following:

- Position yourself at the same level as the patient. Make sure your communication is at the appropriate level for the patient (e.g., little to no medical language, no slang or generational terms).
- Maintain a pleasant facial expression. Sneers, facial expressions of disgust, and other unprofessional facial expressions are signs of disrespect.
- Don't maintain eye contact for too long, because it can be a sign of disrespect. For several cultures, eye contact is disrespectful.
- Use a friendly, professional tone of voice and use words that don't belittle, demean, or purposely make the other person feel uncomfortable.
- Have a friendly, helpful demeanor.
- Refrain from gossiping about patients with co-workers. Not only is it a breach of confidentiality, it also is disrespectful.
- Treat others how you want to be treated.

Scenario: You are a team leader in your department. Your duties include training staff, overseeing student externs, and maintaining the MA work schedule. You work closely with the supervisor and the supervisor talks with you about the problems that Chris is having. Chris is an MA, who has been working in your department for the last 3 months. Several patients have complained about how Chris has talked and acted towards them. They feel talked "down to" and disrespected. The supervisor has noticed a pattern based on the patients complaining. The patients are all "different" from the majority of the patients seen in the department. Your supervisor is upset about the complaints, but more concerned because of the diversity of the patients complaining about Chris. Concerns like this can lead to discrimination lawsuits. Both of you decide that Chris needs to work one-on-one with you as you room patients and interact with patients and families. Chris will be observing how you handle situations where diversity is involved. Through your mentoring, you hope that Chris learns to embrace the diversity and how to respectfully interact with the patients.

Directions for the role-play: To be competent in all areas of this affective competency, the student needs to role-play six different scenarios, selecting one of the two scenarios for each of the six areas. Additional students can be used for the role-play as patient(s) and "Chris."

Diverse Gender

1. A man comes in with a severe case of gynecomastia (enlargement of breast tissue). He is very uncomfortable with the condition.
2. A 21-year-old female comes in with a history of pseudohermaphroditism (the genitalia are of one gender, but some physical characteristics of the other gender are present) and has concerns about her condition, yet she is very uncomfortable discussing it.

Diverse Race

1. An Arab woman comes for an appointment with a female provider. The patient is dressed so that her hair, arms, legs, and body are covered. Your provider requires that all patients change into a gown for the general examination. You know that usually Arab women only uncover areas that need examination and would prefer to remain clothed as much as possible.
2. A Hispanic patient arrives 20 minutes late for an appointment and you are able to work in the patient although it shortens your lunchtime. The patient struggles with speaking English and there is no translator available. Rooming the patient is taking longer than normal.

308

Diverse Religion

1. A female patient who practices Hinduism is your next patient. She needs to see a female provider. When she has come in over the past months, her husband makes all of her healthcare decisions.
2. Your next patient is an 8-day-old boy who needs to have a circumcision today. The parents were insistent the circumcision occurs today since they practice Judaism. Your pediatric provider is held up at the hospital because of an ill child.

Diverse Age

1. You are working in an obstetric department. Your next patient is a 13-year-old middle school girl who is 10 weeks pregnant.
2. You are working in an internal medicine department and your next patient is an 89-year-old gentleman who is hard of hearing and speaks really loud. He likes to talk about the 1950s and how life was prior to technology. You have to redirect him often so you can get his history and obtain his vital signs.

Diverse Economic Status

1. The next patient you are rooming was referred to your clinic from the local free clinic. The patient tells you that she doesn't have any money to pay for her insulin.
2. You are rooming a patient who lives in his car. He appears as if he hasn't had a shower in days.

Diverse Appearance

1. You are working in a pediatric department. Your next patient is a 16-year-old girl who has purple and blue striped hair. She has about six facial piercings and several visible tattoos. Her pants are raggedy and her shirt is tight and low cut. She is chewing gum noisily and gives you minimal answers as you obtain her history.
2. You are working in an internal medicine clinic and your next patient is a 58-year-old male. You call him from the waiting room and notice that he is wearing clothing from the 1960s or 1970s. He has long hair and has a few earrings. His arms are tattooed from his hands to past his elbows.

Scoring Criteria (1 thru 4)	Excellent Evidence of Learning 4	Adequate Evidence of Learning 3	Limited Evidence of Learning 2	Unacceptable Evidence of Learning 1	Score Attempt 1	Score Attempt 2	Score Attempt 3
a. Gender: **Demonstrated respect for individual diversity, including gender, by the use of appropriate verbal and nonverbal communication**	Student demonstrated respect through appropriate body language (e.g., eye contact, facial expressions, gestures) and professional verbal communication (e.g., pleasant, helpful)	Student demonstrated respect through appropriate body language and professional verbal communication, but more practice is needed to look at ease with the patient	Student demonstrated some or limited respectful verbal and/or nonverbal communication behaviors	Student demonstrated a lack of respect for a person who is different; verbal and/or nonverbal communication was disrespectful			
b. Race: **Demonstrated respect for individual diversity, including race, by the use of appropriate verbal and nonverbal communication**	Student demonstrated respect through appropriate body language (e.g., eye contact, facial expressions, gestures) and professional verbal communication (e.g., pleasant, helpful)	Student demonstrated respect through appropriate body language and professional verbal communication, but more practice is needed to look at ease with the patient	Student demonstrated some or limited respectful verbal and/or nonverbal communication behaviors	Student demonstrated a lack of respect for a person who is different; verbal and/or nonverbal communication was disrespectful			

Scoring Criteria (1 thru 4)	Excellent Evidence of Learning 4	Adequate Evidence of Learning 3	Limited Evidence of Learning 2	Unacceptable Evidence of Learning 1	Score Attempt 1	Score Attempt 2	Score Attempt 3
c. Religion: **Demonstrated respect for individual diversity, including religion, by the use of appropriate verbal and nonverbal communication**	Student demonstrated respect through appropriate body language (e.g., eye contact, facial expressions, gestures) and professional verbal communication (e.g., pleasant, helpful)	Student demonstrated respect through appropriate body language and professional verbal communication, but more practice is needed to look at ease with the patient	Student demonstrated some or limited respectful verbal and/or nonverbal communication behaviors	Student demonstrated a lack of respect for a person who is different; verbal and/or nonverbal communication was disrespectful			
d. Age: **Demonstrated respect for individual diversity, including age, by the use of appropriate verbal and nonverbal communication**	Student demonstrated respect through appropriate body language (e.g., eye contact, facial expressions, gestures) and professional verbal communication (e.g., pleasant, helpful)	Student demonstrated respect through appropriate body language and professional verbal communication, but more practice is needed to look at ease with the patient	Student demonstrated some or limited respectful verbal and/or nonverbal communication behaviors	Student demonstrated a lack of respect for a person who is different; verbal and/or nonverbal communication was disrespectful			
e. Economic Status: **Demonstrated respect for individual diversity, including economic status, by the use of appropriate verbal and nonverbal communication**	Student demonstrated respect through appropriate body language (e.g., eye contact, facial expressions, gestures) and professional verbal communication (e.g., pleasant, helpful)	Student demonstrated respect through appropriate body language and professional verbal communication, but more practice is needed to look at ease with the patient	Student demonstrated some or limited respectful verbal and/or nonverbal communication behaviors	Student demonstrated a lack of respect for a person who is different; verbal and/or nonverbal communication was disrespectful			

Scoring Criteria (1 thru 4)	Excellent Evidence of Learning 4	Adequate Evidence of Learning 3	Limited Evidence of Learning 2	Unacceptable Evidence of Learning 1	Score Attempt 1	Score Attempt 2	Score Attempt 3
f. Appearance: **Demonstrated respect for individual diversity, including appearance, by the use of appropriate verbal and nonverbal communication**	Student demonstrated respect through appropriate body language (e.g., eye contact, facial expressions, gestures) and professional verbal communication (e.g., pleasant, helpful)	Student demonstrated respect through appropriate body language and professional verbal communication, but more practice is needed to look at ease with the patient	Student demonstrated some or limited respectful verbal and/or nonverbal communication behaviors	Student demonstrated a lack of respect for a person who is different; verbal and/or nonverbal communication was disrespectful			

Instructor Comments:

PROCEDURE 20-1. PREPARE FOR A STAFF MEETING

CAAHEP COMPETENCIES: V.P.8.
ABHES COMPETENCIES: 7.b., 8.f.

TASK: Prepare for the meeting by creating an agenda and notifying the staff.

EQUIPMENT AND SUPPLIES:
• Computer with word processing software and e-mail
• Paper and pen

Standards: Complete the procedure and all critical steps in _____ minutes with a minimum score of 85% within three attempts.

Scoring: Divide the points earned by the total possible points. Failure to perform a critical step, indicated by an asterisk (*), results in an unsatisfactory overall score.

Time began _____ Time ended _____ Total minutes: _____

Steps	Possible Points	Attempt 1	Attempt 2	Attempt 3
1. Create an agenda using word processing software. Start by listing the attendees, start and end time, and location of the meeting.	10	_____	_____	_____
2. Add the purpose and goal of the meeting.	10	_____	_____	_____
3. Add a list of items to be discussed. The list needs to support or relate to the purpose of the meeting.	10	_____	_____	_____
4. Identify any supplies or materials the attendees should bring to the meeting.	5	_____	_____	_____
*5. Create a professional e-mail to the attendees informing them of the meeting. The e-mail should have an appropriate topic in the subject line. It should include a greeting, appropriate message, and a closing.	25	_____	_____	_____
6. Use correct grammar, spelling, capitalization, and sentence structure in both the agenda and e-mail.	10	_____	_____	_____
7. Proofread both the e-mail and the agenda. Attach the agenda to the e-mail and send the e-mail.	10	_____	_____	_____
8. Create a list of items and equipment needed for the meeting (e.g., whiteboard, easel pad and easel, projector, and computer).	10	_____	_____	_____
9. Create a list of activities you would need to do to prepare for the meeting and to prepare the room for the meeting (e.g., appoint a person to take notes, order food).	10	_____	_____	_____

Comments:

Points earned _____ ÷ 100 possible points = Score _____ % Score

Instructor's signature _____

21 Medical Practice Marketing and Customer Service

VOCABULARY REVIEW

Fill in the blanks with the correct vocabulary terms from the list.

1. Process of informing the local community of the medical procedures and services the healthcare practice provides.
   _____

2. An individual assigned to communicate between multiple parties when the financial responsibilities of a deceased patient's estate are settled. _____

3. Internet-sponsored, two-way communication between individuals, individuals and businesses, or between businesses. _____

4. Video-conferencing technology that enables the delivery of quality healthcare at a distance.
   _____

5. A person who identifies patients' needs and barriers and assists by coordinating care and identifying community and healthcare resources to meet the needs.
   _____

6. Words or graphics on a webpage that, when clicked, take the viewer to another page or another website.
   _____

7. The groups of people most likely to need the medical services the practice offers. _____

8. An online journal that providers can use to share their experiences in caring for patients.
   _____

9. An individual who represents the patient when healthcare decisions are made. _____

10. A model philosophy intended to improve the effectiveness of primary care. This approach is promoted by the National Committee for Quality Assurance (NCQA).
    _____

11. A list of all webpage links on a website.
    _____

12. An assessment that weighs the benefit of attracting patients against the cost required. _____

a. Advocate
b. Blog
c. Cost–benefit analysis
d. Hyperlinks
e. Liaison
f. Marketing
g. Patient-centered medical home (PCMH)
h. Patient navigator
i. Site map
j. Social media
k. Target marketing
l. Telemedicine

Part I: True/False and Multiple Choice
True/False

Indicate whether the statement is true or false. Write your answer on the line.

_____ 1. Marketing can be expensive and ineffective at increasing patient traffic if it is not planned well.

_____ 2. Every dollar spent on marketing will greatly increase patient traffic to the healthcare facility.

_____ 3. Customer service is only important when the patient is in the healthcare agency.

_____ 4. The healthcare facility website traffic should be monitored only during the first three months after the website is created.

_____ 5. The medical assistant should maintain a current list of community resources to assist patients in meeting their healthcare needs.

Multiple Choice

Identify the choice that best completes the statement or answers the question. Write your answer on the line.

_____ 1. Because the medical practice is a business,

    a. New patients are needed to keep the business open long term

    b. The medical practice must charge their patients high prices to stay open

    c. Only interact with patients when they are in the healthcare agency

    d. All extra funds should be spent on marketing

_____ 2. Which of the following marketing strategies costs the least?

    a. A magazine ad

    b. Yearly checkup mailers

    c. Public open house

    d. Managing a social media site

_____ 3. A simple website should have all of the following elements:

    a. Contact Us form

    b. About Us

    c. Patient Testimonials

    d. All of the above

_____ 4. The goal of the patient-centered medical home (PCMH) is to

    a. Improve customer service at healthcare facilities

    b. Recommend patients to community resources

    c. Improve the effectiveness of primary care

    d. Evaluate the effect health insurance coverage has on patient quality of life

_____ 5. Telemedicine is a reflection of what primary healthcare goal?

    a. To recommend patients to community resources

    b. To meet the needs of patients in rural areas

    c. To provide patient care through social media

    d. To provide patient care for those without health insurance

Part II: Short Answers

1. What is meant by "reaching the target market"?

_____

_____

_____

2. What can a healthcare facility do to determine their target market?

_____

_____

3. What information should be kept in a spreadsheet file to determine the demographics of a practice's current patients?

_____

_____

4. What does the acronym SWOT stand for? What is this tool used for?

_____

_____

_____

5. Name five examples of possible strengths a healthcare practice may have over its competitors.

    a. _____

    b. _____

    c. _____

    d. _____

    e. _____

6. Provide five examples of community involvement that may help a medical practice grow.

    a. _____

    b. _____

    c. _____

    d. _____

    e. _____

7. What is the difference between advertising and public relations?

_____

_____

_____

_____

8. What can a healthcare facility do if it receives bad press? Name three possible solutions.

a. _____

b. _____

c. _____

9. List the five basic steps involved in building a website for a medical practice.

a. _____

b. _____

c. _____

d. _____

e. _____

10. Explain why all employees must be committed to providing good customer service.

_____

_____

11. List four phrases and/or body language that should never be used with patients, especially when attempting to provide exceptional customer service.

a. _____

b. _____

c. _____

d. _____

12. In your own words, define patient navigator.

_____

_____

13. Describe the role of the medical assistant as a patient navigator.

_____

_____

14. What are the five key domains of the PCMH model for primary care?

a. _____

b. _____

c. _____

d. _____

e. _____

15. Discuss applications of electronic technology (e.g., telemedicine, video conferencing) in professional communication.

_____

_____

Part III: SWOT Analysis

Review the following case study and perform a SWOT analysis. Complete the figure with at least one item for each category.

The Make Them Feel Better Pediatrics Group has been established in the greater Atlanta metropolitan area for the past eight years. They have three physicians and two nurse practitioners. They operate regular working hours, from 9 AM to 4 PM, Monday through Friday, with a two-hour lunch from 11 AM to 1 PM. About three years ago they moved to electronic health record and practice management software, which increased the efficiency of their processes and saved the staff time. With the increase in efficiency, they were able to open up three more new patient visits and eight additional follow-up visits each week, which allowed them to see more patients.

Over the last several years, the practice has been affected by the Affordable Care Act, which has allowed more people to have health insurance. This created an increase in appointment demands, thus the wait time for appointments has changed from 2 weeks to 2 months. Within the last few weeks, the demand for appointments has increased yet again and it has been attributed to the Atlanta public health department's "Get a Flu Shot" campaign.

Strengths	Weaknesses
Opportunities	Threats

Part IV: Develop a Current List of Community Resources Related to Patients' Healthcare Needs and Facilitate Referrals

For this activity, you will review the scenarios, research local community resources that would be appropriate for the patient, and then role-play providing the patient with the resource list. After the patient decides which resources he or she will use, complete the Community Resource Referral Form. Use a peer for the role-play. Use Procedure 21-1 and Work Product 21-1.

- **Scenario 1:** Herman Miller is a 72-year-old male who was just diagnosed with dementia. He currently lives with his daughter, Ruby, who works full time. Ruby is feeling overwhelmed with being his only caregiver and realizes that she needs to find someone to provide care for her father while she is working.
- **Scenario 2:** Leslie Green just tested positive for pregnancy. She is still a teenager and doesn't feel that she has a support system to help her make decisions.
- **Scenario 3:** Marcia Carrillo's husband of 30 years died suddenly one month ago. Marcia stated that she feels alone and has no one to talk to. Her daughter says that Marcia needs the support of others who have gone through the same thing.

CASE STUDY

Read the case study and answer the question at the end.

Monica, the medical office manager, opens the door to Clear Skin Dermatology at 10 AM and a patient is waiting outside the door. "Good morning," Monica says as she greets the first patient of the day. "Good morning," the patient responds in an irritated tone. "Would you like something to drink? I have some chilled water bottles," Monica asks. "No thank you! It would have been nice for you to notice that I was freezing outside while I was waiting for you to open the door. Why do you open so late, anyway?" sneered the patient.

Monica smiles at the patient and says "My apologies. I was working in the back to prepare for your appointment today and I didn't know you were outside waiting in the cold. It reminds me to keep an eye out for patients in the morning who might be waiting as well. Can I offer you a hot cup of coffee?" The patient feels heard and accepts the coffee and sits patiently waiting to be called.

319

Meanwhile another patient comes in the door. Monica greets her with a friendly "good morning." The patient comes over to the front desk and starts speaking quite loudly about her concerns about how much her insurance will pay for the service she has scheduled today. Monica asks the patient in a soft voice, "Would you like to join me in this private conference room to discuss your concerns and contact the insurance company to find out how much you will be responsible for?" The patient agrees with Monica and follows her to the back conference room.

Later that morning the first patient approached Monica praising her for their interaction earlier. The patient admitted that she had not had her coffee yet and may have been a little grouchy. Monica takes the opportunity to accept the praise and encourages the patient to complete a simple 5-minute survey before she left. The patient was happy to comply! Monica also encouraged the patient to visit the Clear Skin Dermatology Facebook page to share her positive experience.

1. Describe the three different instances where Monica provided high-quality customer service.

   _____

2. If you were working with Monica, what additional ways could you provide exceptional customer service?

   _____

WORKPLACE APPLICATION

Complete this activity and share your results with the class, if appropriate.

Providing exceptional customer service can actually interfere with job duties. Some workers use customer service as an excuse to chat with patients and avoid other duties. Determine how the medical assistant can strike a balance between providing the customer service that patients deserve and completing all the tasks required each day.

INTERNET ACTIVITIES

Complete one or more of these activities and share your results with the class, if appropriate.

1. Research customer service and develop your own original definition of the concept of customer service. Present your thoughts to the class by creating a professional presentation.

2. Research public relations and make a list of the various "free" ways that publicity can be generated for the office. Choose five ideas you feel are the best. E-mail these ideas to each of your classmates.

3. Research the patient navigator position and duties. Summarize your findings.

4. Create a fictional medical clinic and explain how social media could be used to enhance its web presence. Provide examples of specific ways in which social media would drive patients to use the website or the actual facility.

PROCEDURE 21-1. DEVELOP A CURRENT LIST OF COMMUNITY RESOURCES RELATED TO PATIENTS' HEALTHCARE NEEDS AND FACILITATE REFERRALS

MAERB/CAAHEP COMPETENCIES: V.P.9., V.P.10.
ABHES COMPETENCIES: 5.b.3., 8.f.

TASK: Create a list of appropriate community resources related to patients' healthcare needs to facilitate referrals to community resources in the role of a patient navigator.

EQUIPMENT AND SUPPLIES:
- Computer with Internet and/or a telephone book
- Paper and pen
- Community Resource Referral Form (Work Product 21-1) or referral form

Standards: Complete the Procedure and all critical steps in _____ minutes with a minimum score of 85% within three attempts.

Scoring: Divide the points earned by the total possible points. Failure to perform a critical step, indicated by an asterisk (*), results in an unsatisfactory overall score.

Time began _____ Time ended _____ Total minutes: _____

Steps	Possible Points	Attempt 1	Attempt 2	Attempt 3
1. Identify the types of community resources that might assist the patient and/or family.	20	_____	_____	_____
2. Using the Internet and/or the phone book, identify local resources for the patient. Make a list of resources for the patient and/or family member. Include the name of the organization, the address, and the contact information.	30	_____	_____	_____
3. Summarize the services provided by the organization.	20	_____	_____	_____
4. (Role-play) Provide the patient and/or family member with the list of resources and identify the service(s) that would interest them.	10	_____	_____	_____
5. Use professional, tactful verbal and nonverbal communication as you work with the patient and family.	10	_____	_____	_____
6. Complete the referral form to help facilitate the referral to community resource(s).	10	_____	_____	_____

Comments:

Points earned _____ ÷ 100 possible points = Score _____ % Score

Instructor's signature _____

Name: _____ Date: _____

WORK PRODUCT 21-1. COMMUNITY RESOURCE REFERRAL FORM

Corresponds to PROCEDURE 21-1

MAERB/CAAHEP COMPETENCIES: V.P.9., V.P.10.
ABHES COMPETENCIES: 5.b.3., 8.f.

Patient's Name:	Date of Birth:

Community Resource Information:

Agency: _____ Contact Name: _____

Address: _____ Phone number: _____

_____ Website: _____

Services Provided:	

Agency: _____ Contact Name: _____

Address: _____ Phone number: _____

_____ Website: _____

Services Provided:	

Agency: _____ Contact Name: _____

Address: _____ Phone number: _____

_____ Website: _____

Services Provided:	

Agency: _____ Contact Name: _____

Address: _____ Phone number: _____

_____ Website: _____

Services Provided:	

323

22 Safety and Emergency Practices

VOCABULARY REVIEW

Define the following terms.

1. Cyanosis

2. Diaphoresis

3. Ecchymosis

4. Emetic

5. Fibrillation

6. Hematuria

7. Mediastinum

8. Myocardium

9. Necrosis

10. Photophobia

11. Polydipsia

12. Thrombolytics

13. Transient ischemic attack

_____

Fill in the blanks with the correct terms.

14. _____ is defined as the immediate care given to a person who has been injured or has suddenly become ill.

15. AED stands for _____.

16. CPR stands for _____.

17. CVA is a(n) _____.

18. TIA is a(n) _____.

19. Myocardial infarction is a(n) _____.

20. SDS are _____.

21. _____ is the most dangerous form of heat-related injury and results in a shutdown of body systems.

22. _____ are the initial signs of a heat-related emergency.

23. Patients with _____ appear flushed and report headaches, nausea, vertigo, and weakness.

24. If the physician diagnoses a disease that has no known cause, it is called _____.

SKILLS AND CONCEPTS

1. Summarize a minimum of four methods of maintaining a safe environment for both staff and patients.

   a. _____

   b. _____

   c. _____

   d. _____

2. Identify five methods for preventing fires in the ambulatory care center.

   a. _____

   b. _____

   c. _____

   d. _____

   e. _____

3. Explain the procedure for effectively discharging a fire extinguisher.

   _____

   _____

   _____

4. Describe the fundamental principles for evacuation of a healthcare setting.

_____

_____

_____

_____

5. List and define the four levels of evacuation that should be followed if there is an emergency in the facility.

_____

_____

_____

_____

6. Ambulatory care providers should be prepared to contact community emergency services as needed. Identify five resources available in your community for emergency preparedness. Include the services provided and contact information for each.

a. _____

b. _____

c. _____

d. _____

e. _____

7. Standard precautions are crucial for preventing the transmission of diseases associated with bioterrorism. Summarize infection control procedures that should be implemented in the event a bioterrorism incident may have occurred.

_____

_____

_____

8. Explain the purpose of the Laboratory Response Network.

_____

_____

_____

9. Summarize the recommendations of the Centers for Disease Control and Prevention (CDC) to help minimize the negative psychological effects of an emergency situation on both staff members and patients.

_____

_____

_____

_____

_____

10. The Occupational Safety and Health Administration (OSHA) recommends multiple factors that can help promote staff safety. Explain six accident prevention behaviors that should be followed in a healthcare setting.

a. _____

b. _____

c. _____

d. _____

e. _____

f. _____

11. You are responsible for placing and labeling biohazard waste containers in the provider's office where you work. Explain the protocols for the proper disposal of biologic chemic material in a healthcare setting.

_____

_____

_____

_____

12. Discuss the role of medical assistants in emergency preparedness and the ways they can help if a natural disaster or other emergency occurs in their community.

_____

_____

_____

_____

_____

13. List five symptoms of a heart attack.

a. _____

b. _____

c. _____

d. _____

e. _____

14. What are the myocardial signs and symptoms that may be experienced by female patients?

_____

_____

_____

15. List and explain seven types of shock.

   a. _____

   b. _____

   c. _____

   d. _____

   e. _____

   f. _____

   g. _____

16. Summarize the FAST guidelines developed by the American Stroke Association to help people spot the signs of a sudden stroke.

   _____

   _____

   _____

   _____

17. Explain the differences between sprains and strains.

   _____

   _____

   _____

18. Give two examples of situations in which patients with abdominal pain should be seen by a healthcare provider immediately.

   a. _____

   b. _____

19. Explain how a patient in shock should be managed.

   _____

   _____

   _____

20. Screening emergency telephone calls is an important role of the medical assistant in the ambulatory care setting. List a minimum of two questions the medical assistant should ask for the following health problems.

   a. Syncope (fainting)

   _____

   _____

   b. Head injury

   _____

   _____

   _____

c. Insect bites or stings

_____

_____

d. Burns

_____

_____

e. Wounds

_____

_____

f. Animal bites

_____

_____

g. Asthma

_____

_____

h. Poisoning

_____

_____

21. Identify critical elements of an emergency plan for response to a natural disaster or other emergency.

_____

_____

_____

_____

_____

_____

CASE STUDIES

Read the case studies and answer the questions that follow.

1. Sally calls the office complaining of abdominal pain that has been present for the past 2 days. What type of screening questions should you ask the patient? When should the patient be seen in the office? Provide the appropriate documentation.

_____

_____

_____

2. Mr. Walker, a 64-year-old patient, calls the office complaining of shortness of breath, pressure in the chest, and sweating for the past hour. Upon checking the patient's record, you find that Mr. Walker is a smoker and obese. How should you manage this call? Show your documentation.

_____

_____

_____

3. The provider refers Mr. Walker to the emergency department, but he refuses to go, stating, "I don't feel well enough to drive to the hospital." What should be done to meet the needs of the patient? Document your conversation.

_____

_____

_____

4. A patient calls, stating that she has found a tick on her left forearm. Explain the proper technique for removal of the tick. Should the provider see this patient? Document your conversation.

_____

_____

_____

5. A 19-year-old patient sitting in the waiting room experiences a grand mal seizure. What should Cheryl, the medical assistant, do to prevent injury to the patient? After the seizure, the patient needs to be placed in the recovery position to maintain her airway. Explain how to place her in this position.

_____

_____

_____

6. The mother of a 10-year-old child comes running into the office with her son. He is bleeding profusely from a gash in his left forearm. She states he fell on some glass at the playground and she just rushed him to the physician's office. What should be done immediately to control the bleeding from the wound? Include in your discussion OSHA precautions for possible contamination.

_____

_____

_____

WORKPLACE APPLICATION OPTIONS

Complete one or more of these activities and, if appropriate, share your results with the class.

1. The school you attend has automated external defibrillators available in each building. Describe to the students in your class how to use one in a cardiac emergency.

_____

_____

_____

_____

2. You learned in your text about factors that are crucial for patient safety and a few of the most common mistakes that can be made by healthcare workers that result in injury to a patient. Develop a handout that summarizes patient safety factors and share it with the class.

3. Dr. Bendt orders you to start 2 LPM of oxygen on a patient with complaints of shortness of breath (SOB). Explain how you would perform this task and what should be documented in the patient's health record.

_____

_____

_____

_____

4. At a recent office meeting, telephone screening difficulties were addressed. Dr. Bendt asks you to review the current procedures and policies that are followed when patients call the office with emergencies and offer suggestions on how possible questions might be improved. In addition, the physician would like you to make a list of "home care advice" to go along with the symptoms. The work should also include "if" and "how soon" the patient should be seen in the office or under what circumstances the patient should be referred to the emergency department. Include the following situations in your project.

Asthma	Insect bites and stings
Wounds	Head injuries
Burns	Chest pain
Animal bites	Hypoglycemia
Fractures	Hyperglycemia
Poisoning	Syncope

5. As a medical assistant, you understand that medical emergencies have many different signs and symptoms. Dr. Bendt has asked you to create an informative brochure to educate patients about the problem. Choose a topic discussed in the chapter and create a handout that includes the following:

   a. Definition of illness or injury

   b. Importance of early detection

   c. Signs and symptoms

   d. Risk factors

   e. Prevention recommendations

   f. What patients should do if they think they are experiencing this condition

6. Refer to the illustration in your text that shows pictures of OSHA's recommended formats for safety signs, symbols, and labels. These should be posted in the ambulatory care setting to warn patients of potential danger or to help with evacuation of the facility in an emergency. Search for these signs in your practice laboratory at your school as well as in the building where your classes are held. Refer to Procedure 22-1. Is your school in compliance?

_____

_____

_____

7. Cheryl is in charge of maintaining the office crash cart. What type of supplies should be stocked in the cart? What medications should be included?

_____

_____

_____

_____

_____

_____

8. The medical assistant can play an integral role in a community's response to natural or human-created disasters. Summarize how the medical assistant can contribute to the community response to an emergency.

_____

_____

_____

_____

9. The daughter of an elderly stroke victim is very concerned about her father's potential for choking. Explain to the daughter what to do if her father experiences an obstructed airway. Include in your explanation the techniques for both responsive and unresponsive adults.

_____

_____

_____

_____

INTERNET ACTIVITY OPTIONS

Complete one or more of these activities and, if appropriate, share your results with the class.

1. You notice that your CPR for the professional certification is about to expire. Search for a list of certification sites in your area. Make a list of the contact information and share the locations with your classmates.

2. Perform a search for the poison control center in your area. Search for and create a list of ideas for ways to prevent poisoning. Create an informative poster to display in your physician's office.

3. Investigate the CDC site for emergency preparedness planning at www.bt.cdc.gov/planning/#healthcare.

4. Search the CDC Emergency Operations Center site at www.cdc.gov/phpr/eoc.htm. What is the responsibility of the EOC?

HEALTH RECORD ACTIVITIES

Documentation of an onsite emergency includes the following information:

- Patient's name, address, age, and health insurance information
- Allergies, current medications, and pertinent health history
- Name and relationship of any person with the patient
- Vital signs and chief complaint
- Sequence of events, beginning with how the problem occurred, any changes in the patient's overall condition, and any observations made regarding the patient's condition
- Details of procedures or treatments performed on the patient

Document the details of the following cases.

1. Charise Mourning calls at 4 PM, just after the physician has left for the day, and reports that her husband, Sam, fell going down the steps and can't bear weight on his left leg. Mrs. Mourning is 78 years old and does not know how to drive. What questions should you ask? How should you handle the situation? Document pertinent information in Mr. Mourning's health record.

_____

_____

_____

_____

_____

2. Lynne Franklin, the 17-year-old mother of a 9-month-old son, calls, hysterical and crying. She states that the baby is "jerking and shaking all over the crib." She states, "I tried to hold him down, and I heard something snap! What should I do? He looks like he is turning blue!" Lynne tells you he had a fever all night. The last time she took his temperature it was 103° F axillary. She is alone with the baby. How should the situation be handled? Document the details in the baby's health record.

_____

_____

_____

_____

3. Charles Drysden, a 42-year-old patient, calls when the rest of the office is out to lunch. He is at work and is experiencing heaviness in his chest, difficulty breathing, indigestion, sweating, and minor jaw discomfort. He reports that the discomfort in his chest started about 30 minutes ago, after he ate a large lunch. Mr. Drysden took Mylanta for the indigestion but is not feeling any better. He wants to drive himself to the office even though a co-worker has offered to take him to the emergency department (ED). His pain is getting worse, but he doesn't think he needs to go to the ED. What should you do? Document the important details in Mr. Drysden's health record.

_____

_____

_____

_____

4. A patient enters the waiting room accompanied by his girlfriend without an appointment. He is holding his right arm and is in obvious distress. He tells you he fell during a softball game and heard something snap in his wrist. The provider orders you to apply a splint to the patient's wrist before he is transported to the emergency department. Explain the steps in applying a splint to a possible fracture. Document the procedure in the patient's health record.

_____

_____

_____

_____

5. The wife of a patient calls early one morning to report her husband is "acting strange." The patient has diabetes, and the wife cannot tell you if he took his insulin this morning or if he has eaten anything since last night. What is the initial recommendation for managing a diabetic emergency? The patient has a glucometer at home, and his wife knows how to use it. What should you ask her to do? If the blood glucose level is below 80 and the patient is able to swallow, what is the recommendation?

_____

_____

_____

_____

_____

6. You are working in the administrative area of the office when a patient enters the waiting room screaming for attention. She insists the physician ordered the wrong medication, and she wants to talk to the doctor immediately. The physician is not in the office today, so you attempt to handle this very angry patient. Using the skills discussed in Procedure 22-2: Manage a Difficult Patient, try to work out a solution with the patient. Document the patient interaction in the woman's health record.

_____

_____

_____

_____

_____

AFFECTIVE COMPETENCIES: XII.A.1. RECOGNIZE THE PHYSICAL AND EMOTIONAL EFFECTS ON PERSONS INVOLVED IN AN EMERGENCY SITUATION

Student name _____ Date_____

Explanation: Student must achieve a minimum score of 3 in each category to achieve competency.

Psychological Aspects of an Emergency Situation

A wide variety of stress-related behaviors are seen in patients experiencing an emergency situation. These include a change in appetite, feeling powerless, withdrawal from social interaction, and sleep difficulties. In addition, everyone involved in an emergency situation experiences a certain amount of anxiety and stress. The medical assistant should use therapeutic communications—restatement, reflection, and clarification—and appropriate body language to help gather information during an emergency situation and reassure patients as well as staff.

The CDC recommends that a facility's emergency preparedness plan consider the following steps to minimize these negative psychological effects on both healthcare workers and patients:

- Provide fact sheets for employees and patients to help them understand the dangers of certain emergencies and encourage employee participation in disaster drills.
- Plan in advance for effective communication and action in response to an emergency; the plan should include methods for coordinating a response with local and state agencies and media sources.
- Put into place a method for clearly explaining emergency situations to patients and healthcare workers; offer immediate evaluation and treatment of an infectious outbreak.
- Treat acute anxiety with reassurance and explanation; provide follow-up counseling as needed for employees.

Using the following case studies role-play with your partner how you would recognize the effects of stress in those involved in emergency situations.

The mother of an acutely ill young child is extremely upset about her child's condition. She is unable to focus on the details of treatment and cannot stop crying. Demonstrate how you would manage this situation.

There are reports of a shooting at a mall close to where you work. One of the staff members becomes extremely upset because her sister works in the mall. She falls to the floor screaming and crying and wants to leave immediately to check on her sister. There are patients in the office, and the physician decides to continue providing care for patients who are present. Demonstrate how you would manage this situation.

Scoring Criteria (1 to 4)	Excellent Evidence of Learning 4	Adequate Evidence of Learning 3	Limited Evidence of Learning 2	Unacceptable Evidence of Learning 1	Score Attempt 1	Score Attempt 2	Score Attempt 3
Recognizes the physical and emotional effects on persons involved in an emergency situation	Student demonstrates the highest level of awareness of the physical and emotional effects on persons involved in emergency situations	Student demonstrates mastery level of awareness of the physical and emotional effects on persons involved in emergency situations	Student is developing competency in awareness of the physical and emotional effects on persons involved in emergency situations	Student inadequately demonstrates the main concepts of the physical and emotional effects on persons involved in emergency situations			

Scoring Criteria (1 to 4)	Excellent Evidence of Learning 4	Adequate Evidence of Learning 3	Limited Evidence of Learning 2	Unacceptable Evidence of Learning 1	Score Attempt 1	Score Attempt 2	Score Attempt 3
Recognizes the importance of patient/staff socioeconomic status, age, gender, race, religion, educational level, and cultural experience in terms of how they react to an emergency situation	Correctly identifies the effect of individual diversity on the response to emergency situations	Recognizes some of the effect of individual diversity on the response to emergency situations, but the approach is not comprehensive	Shows limited recognition of the effect of individual diversity on the response to emergency situations	Fails to recognize the effect of individual diversity on the response to emergency situations			
Analyzes the individual's physical and emotional response to an emergency situation and makes a decision on how to help	Considers all of the individual factors affecting persons involved in an emergency situation before reaching a solution	Identifies most of the individual factors affecting persons involved in an emergency situation before reaching a solution	Shows limited recognition of individual factors affecting persons involved in an emergency situation before reaching a solution	Fails to identify significant individual factors affecting persons involved in an emergency situation before reaching a solution			
Evaluates the outcome of the response to an emergency situation	Assesses the outcome of the response to an emergency situation	Briefly considers the outcome of the response to an emergency situation	Shows limited consideration of the outcome of the response to an emergency situation	Fails to evaluate the outcome of the response to an emergency situation			

Instructor comments:

AFFECTIVE COMPETENCIES: XII.A.2. DEMONSTRATE SELF-AWARENESS IN RESPONDING TO EMERGENCY SITUATIONS

Student name _____ Date_____

Explanation: Student must achieve a minimum score of 3 in each category to achieve competency.

Ambulatory care centers and hospitals may be the first to recognize and initiate a response to a community emergency. Every healthcare facility should have a policy with specific procedures for the management of emergencies on site. When a new employee starts on the job, part of the orientation process is to review the site's policy and procedures manual. As a new employee, be sure to clarify any questions you have about emergency management in that particular facility.

Staff members should discuss possible emergencies that may occur and should have an emergency action plan for rapid, systematic intervention. For instance, local industries may present unique problems that call for very specialized care. Plan for these and ask the physician's advice on the procedures to follow and the supplies to have on hand. If the facility has several employees, each should be assigned specific duties in the event of an emergency. Organization and planning make the difference between systematic care for patients and complete chaos.

Medical emergencies can happen at any time in an ambulatory care center. The medical assistant may be responsible for initiating first aid and continuing to administer it until the physician or trained medical team arrives. Medical assistants are not responsible for diagnosing emergencies, especially over the telephone, but they are expected to make decisions about emergency situations based on their medical knowledge and training. If any doubt exists about how to manage a particular situation or emergency phone call, the medical assistant should not hesitate to consult the physician, the office manager, or some other more experienced member of the healthcare team.

The Medical Assistant's Role in Performing Emergency Procedures
- Perform only the emergency procedures for which you have been trained.
- If an emergency occurs in the facility, notify the physician.
- If a physician cannot be located, immediately contact the local EMS team.

Using the following case study role-play with your partner how you would demonstrate self-awareness in responding to the following emergency situation.

There are reports of a shooting at a close to where you work. The office manager explains support staff is needed to help with the care of survivors and implements the facility's environmental disaster plan. You are sent to the emergency triage site to assist with victims, and your partner is expected to help evacuate the facility. Demonstrate how you would manage this situation.

Scoring Criteria (1 to 4)	Excellent Evidence of Learning 4	Adequate Evidence of Learning 3	Limited Evidence of Learning 2	Unacceptable Evidence of Learning 1	Score Attempt 1	Score Attempt 2	Score Attempt 3
Student demonstrates self-awareness in responding to emergency situations	Student demonstrates the highest level of self-awareness in responding to emergency situations	Student demonstrates mastery level of self-awareness in responding to emergency situations	Student is developing competency in self-awareness in responding to emergency situations	Student demonstrates the main concepts of self-awareness in responding to emergency situations, but does not implement strategies adequately			

Scoring Criteria (1 to 4)	Excellent Evidence of Learning 4	Adequate Evidence of Learning 3	Limited Evidence of Learning 2	Unacceptable Evidence of Learning 1	Score Attempt 1	Score Attempt 2	Score Attempt 3
Student responds to the emergency situation appropriately	Student demonstrates an appropriate and correct response to his or her role in the management of the emergency situation	Student demonstrates an appropriate response to his or her role in the management of the emergency situation, but the approach is not comprehensive	Student demonstrates a limited response to his or her role in the management of the emergency situation	Student fails to demonstrate an appropriate and correct response to his or her role in the management of the emergency situation			

Instructor comments:

PROCEDURE 22-1. EVALUATE THE WORK ENVIRONMENT TO IDENTIFY UNSAFE WORKING CONDITIONS AND COMPLY WITH SAFETY SIGNS AND SYMBOLS

CAAHEP COMPETENCIES: XII.P.1.a-c., XII.P.5.
ABHES COMPETENCIES: 9.g.

TASK: Assess the healthcare facility for possible safety issues and develop a safety plan.

SCENARIO: Work with a partner to evaluate environmental safety in the laboratory at your school. Record your results and discuss with the class. After the class members share their observations, develop a safety plan for your laboratory.

EQUIPMENT AND SUPPLIES:
• Pen and paper
• Document or manual on policies and procedures for environmental safety issues in the facility

Standards: Complete the procedure and all critical steps in _____ minutes with a minimum score of 85% in three attempts.

Scoring: Divide the points earned by the total possible points. All steps in this procedure are considered critical. Failure to perform a single critical step results in an unsatisfactory overall score.

Time began _____ Time ended _____ Total minutes: _____

Steps	Possible Points	Attempt 1	Attempt 2	Attempt 3
1. Check the floors and hallways for obstructions and possible tripping hazards, including torn carpets, possible spills, protruding electrical cords, and so on.	6	_____	_____	_____
2. Check storage areas to make sure the tops of cabinets are clear and heavier items are stored closer to the floor.	6	_____	_____	_____
3. Assess the location and security of handrails and grab bars placed around the facility. They should be placed with all stairs, in bathrooms, and in any other areas staff members or patients may need assistance.	6	_____	_____	_____
4. Examine all electrical plugs and outlets to prevent electrical overload.	6	_____	_____	_____
5. Check all equipment to make sure it is in safe working condition.	10	_____	_____	_____
6. Make sure all lights are working (both inside and outside the facility), that lighting is adequate, and that light fixtures are in good condition.	10	_____	_____	_____
7. Check the working condition of smoke alarms and examine all fire extinguishers.	10	_____	_____	_____
8. Make sure evacuation routes are posted throughout the facility, with clearly marked exit routes and floor plans with exits marked.	10	_____	_____	_____

341

Steps	Possible Points	Attempt 1	Attempt 2	Attempt 3
9. Assess the laboratory's compliance with the safety signs, symbols, and labels required by the Occupational Safety and Health Administration (OSHA). Are all signs, symbols, labels in place and posted properly?	16			
a. Refrigerators used for storage of medical supplies and specimens are labeled with a biohazard symbol and bear the legend "not for storage of food or medications."		_____	_____	_____
b. Biohazard waste receptacles have the biohazard symbol and are lined with red plastic bags.		_____	_____	_____
c. Chemicals and reagents are evaluated for hazard category classification and labeled with the National Fire Association's color and number coding.		_____	_____	_____
d. Signs are clearly posted in appropriate places for prohibiting smoking, eating, drinking, or application of cosmetics or contact lenses in the facility.		_____	_____	_____
10. Record your observations and share them with the class.	10	_____	_____	_____
11. Based on group discussion, develop a plan of action for improving the safety of the laboratory.	10	_____	_____	_____

Comments:

Points earned _____ ÷ 100 possible points = **Score** _____ **% Score**

Instructor's signature _____

Name _____ Date _____ Score _____

PROCEDURE 22-2. MANAGE A DIFFICULT PATIENT

CAAHEP COMPETENCIES: XII.P.5.
ABHES COMPETENCIES: 9.g.

TASK: Role-play communication with an angry patient in a safe, therapeutic manner. The following procedure is part of an overall employee safety plan.

SCENARIO: You are working at the admissions desk when an extremely angry patient comes storming into the office, yelling about a mistake on his bill. Although the facility uses an outside billing center, you recognize that you should try to help the patient and attempt to defuse the situation. *Remember:* Call 911 immediately and alert any available security if you or one of your co-workers is threatened with violence.

EQUIPMENT AND SUPPLIES:
• Patient's record
• Telephone
• Facility's policies and procedures manual

Standards: Complete the procedure and all critical steps in _____ minutes with a minimum score of 85% in three attempts.

Scoring: Divide the points earned by the total possible points. Failure to perform a critical step, indicated by an asterisk (*), results in an unsatisfactory overall score.

Time began _____ **Time ended** _____ **Total minutes:** _____

Steps	Possible Points	Attempt 1	Attempt 2	Attempt 3
*1. Although it is important to safeguard a patient's privacy, do not ask an angry patient into an isolated room; do not close the door.	10	_____	_____	_____
2. Alert other staff members to the situation, if possible.	10	_____	_____	_____
3. If you do not feel physically threatened, allow the patient to blow off steam.	10	_____	_____	_____
*4. When the patient begins to slow down, offer supportive statements, such as, "I understand it is frustrating to receive a bill you think is unfair." Continue to make supportive statements until the patient is calmer (think of it as the patient screaming his way up a mountain; sooner or later he is going to run out of steam; when he begins to slow down, you can then start offering supportive statements).	15	_____	_____	_____
*5. Once you can discuss the situation, ask the patient for the details of the problem. Gather as much information as possible so that you can work together on a possible solution.	20	_____	_____	_____
*6. After determining the problem, suggest a possible solution. For example, you will contact the billing office with the information and make sure they get back to the patient as soon as possible.	15	_____	_____	_____

Steps	Possible Points	Attempt 1	Attempt 2	Attempt 3
7. Report the incident to your supervisor and document the patient's problem and the agreed-upon action in the patient's health record, taking care not to use judgmental statements.	10	_____	_____	_____
8. Discuss your approach to managing the difficult patient at the next staff meeting. With your supervisort's permission, summarize your approach and include it as part of the facilityt's Employee Safety Plan.	10	_____	_____	_____

Documentation in the Health Record

Comments:

Points earned _____ ÷ 100 possible points = **Score** _____ **% Score**

Instructor's signature _____

Name _____ Date _____ Score _____

PROCEDURE 22-3. DEMONSTRATE THE PROPER USE OF A FIRE EXTINGUISHER

CAAHEP COMPETENCIES: XII.P.2.b.
ABHES COMPETENCIES: 9.g.

TASK: Role-play the safe and proper use of a fire extinguisher.

EQUIPMENT AND SUPPLIES:
• Portable, office-size ABC fire extinguisher that has been discharged

Standards: Complete the procedure and all critical steps in _____ minutes with a minimum score of 85% in three attempts.

Scoring: Divide the points earned by the total possible points. All steps are critical to the completion of this procedure. Failure to perform a single critical step will result in an unsatisfactory overall score.

Time began _____ Time ended _____ Total minutes: _____

Steps	Possible Points	Attempt 1	Attempt 2	Attempt 3
1. Pull the pin from the handle of the extinguisher.	20	_____	_____	_____
2. Aim the discharge from the extinguisher toward the bottom of the flames.	20	_____	_____	_____
3. Squeeze the handle of the extinguisher so that it begins to discharge.	20	_____	_____	_____
4. Sweep the extinguisher from side to side toward the base of the fire until it is out or until fire officials arrive.	20	_____	_____	_____
5. Check on the safety of all patients and other personnel.	20	_____	_____	_____

Comments:

Points earned _____ ÷ 100 possible points = **Score** _____ **% Score**

Instructor's signature _____

PROCEDURE 22-4. PARTICIPATE IN A MOCK ENVIRONMENTAL EXPOSURE EVENT: EVACUATE A PROVIDER'S OFFICE

CAAHEP COMPETENCIES: XII.P.4.
ABHES COMPETENCIES: 9.g.

TASK: Role-play an environmental disaster and implement an evacuation plan.

SCENARIO: Role-play this scenario with your laboratory group: The building next door to the provider's office where you work is on fire. One member of the group is the designated emergency action coordinator, two individuals are responsible for helping patients with special needs out of the facility, and one person is designated to be the last to leave after the building has been cleared. In a community emergency situation, certain staff members may be designated to provide immediate assistance to survivors. Two medical assistants are sent to help with fire victims. After the evacuation is complete, meet in a designated spot to discuss the process and determine whether the evacuation plan could be improved in any areas. Document the steps taken throughout the mock environmental event.

EQUIPMENT AND SUPPLIES:
- Pen and paper
- Document or manual on policies and procedures for evacuation of the facility and response to an environmental disaster

Standards: Complete the procedure and all critical steps in _____ minutes with a minimum score of 85% in three attempts.

Scoring: Divide the points earned by the total possible points. Failure to perform a critical step, indicated by an asterisk (*), results in an unsatisfactory overall score.

Time began _____ Time ended _____ Total minutes: _____

Steps	Possible Points	Attempt 1	Attempt 2	Attempt 3
*1. An emergency action coordinator is put in charge. The student who is role-playing the emergency action coordinator takes action to manage the emergency at the facility and notifies and works with community emergency services.	5	_____	_____	_____
*2. Victims of the fire are being cared for across the street, where a triage and treatment center has been set up by the city's police, fire, and emergency responder units. Two students role-play staff members who are sent to help. They do the following:				
a. Use therapeutic communication techniques to calm and care for victims.	3	_____	_____	_____
b. Implement appropriate Standard Precautions.	3	_____	_____	_____
c. Monitor and record vital signs.	3	_____	_____	_____
d. Gather pertinent health histories.	3	_____	_____	_____
e. Observe victims for possible complications (e.g., breathing problems, shock, angina).	3	_____	_____	_____
f. Immediately report any life-threatening changes in a patient's status to emergency responders.	3	_____	_____	_____
g. Use first aid skills as needed.	3	_____	_____	_____

347

Steps	Possible Points	Attempt 1	Attempt 2	Attempt 3
*3. The coordinator designates an employee to shut down immediately any combustibles (e.g., oxygen tanks).	10	_____	_____	_____
*4. Using the posted evacuation routes, role-play staff members follow floor plan diagrams to the closest safe exit. They also identify any hazardous areas in the facility to avoid during the emergency evacuation. Role-play staff members assisting patients, especially those with special needs (e.g., individuals in wheelchairs) during the building evacuation.	10	_____	_____	_____
*5. Role-play the staff member delegated to check that everyone has left the facility and that fire doors have been closed before he or she leaves the building.	10	_____	_____	_____
*6. Role-play evacuated personnel and patients meeting in a designated area to count heads and make sure everyone exited the facility safely.	10	_____	_____	_____
*7. After everyone has been accounted for and patients are safe, role-play staff members reporting to the emergency triage area to provide assistance to rescue workers and victims.	10	_____	_____	_____
8. Discuss the evacuation exercise and response to a community disaster with the class.	10	_____	_____	_____
*9. Document the specific steps taken during the facility evacuation and your role in the exercise. What were the strengths and weaknesses of the group's response to an environmental emergency?	14	_____	_____	_____

Assess and document your role in the exercise:

Comments:

Points earned _____ ÷ 100 possible points = **Score** _____ **% Score**

Instructor's signature _____

Name _____ Date _____ Score _____

PROCEDURE 22-5. MAINTAIN AN UP-TO-DATE LIST OF COMMUNITY RESOURCES FOR EMERGENCY PREPAREDNESS

CAAHEP COMPETENCIES: V.P.9.
ABHES COMPETENCIES: 9.i.

TASK: Role-play the following scenario and develop a list of community resources that would respond to a natural disaster or other emergency.

SCENARIO: You are asked by your employer to develop a list of groups in your community that are part of the community-wide emergency preparedness plan mandated by the state and federal government. Using multiple resources, develop a comprehensive list of emergency services for your area.

EQUIPMENT AND SUPPLIES:
- Telephone
- Internet access
- Pen and paper
- Electronic record

Standards: Complete the procedure and all critical steps in _____ minutes with a minimum score of 85% in three attempts.

Scoring: Divide the points earned by the total possible points. All steps in this procedure are considered critical. Failure to perform a single critical step results in an unsatisfactory overall score.

Time began _____ **Time ended** _____ **Total minutes:** _____

Steps	Possible Points	Attempt 1	Attempt 2	Attempt 3
1. Start with an online search for the area office of the Local Emergency Management Agency (LEMA), which is sponsored by the Department of Homeland Security. If available, investigate the LEMA website for information about the emergency preparedness plan in your community. You can begin the search at the website *www.ready.gov*; the Federal Emergency Management Agency (FEMA) website is *www.fema.gov*.	25	_____	_____	_____
2. Gather contact information for local police, fire, and emergency medical services (EMS); post this information next to all telephones in the facility.	25	_____	_____	_____
3. Investigate services provided by your local Public Health office and the American Red Cross.	25	_____	_____	_____
4. Organize the information you gathered about community resources for emergency preparedness. With your instructor's approval, post a copy of this information in all appropriate locations in the facility. Prepare a database in the computer that can be updated as the information changes.	25	_____	_____	_____

Comments:

Points earned _____ ÷ 100 possible points = Score _____ % Score

Instructor's signature _____

Name _____ Date _____ Score _____

PROCEDURE 22-6. MAINTAIN PROVIDER/PROFESSIONAL-LEVEL CPR CERTIFICATION: USE AN AUTOMATED EXTERNAL DEFIBRILLATOR (AED)

CAAHEP COMPETENCIES: I.P.12.
ABHES COMPETENCIES: 9.g.

TASK: Defibrillate adult victims with cardiac arrest. Most adult victims in sudden cardiac arrest are in ventricular fibrillation. The survival rate for victims with ventricular fibrillation is as high as 90% when defibrillation occurs within the first minute of collapse; however, the survival rate declines 7% to 10% with every minute defibrillation does not occur.

EQUIPMENT AND SUPPLIES:
- Practice automated external defibrillator (AED)
- Approved mannequin

Standards: Complete the procedure and all critical steps in _____ minutes with a minimum score of 85% in three attempts.

Scoring: Divide the points earned by the total possible points. All steps in this procedure are considered critical. Failure to perform a single critical step results in an unsatisfactory overall score.

Time began _____ **Time ended** _____ **Total minutes:** _____
These steps are to be performed only on an approved mannequin with a practice AED.
 If the healthcare worker witnesses a cardiac arrest, an AED should be used as soon as possible. If CPR has already been started, continue performing CPR until the AED machine is turned on, pads are applied, and the machine is ready.

Steps	Possible Points	Attempt 1	Attempt 2	Attempt 3
1. Place the AED near the victim's left ear and then turn on the machine.	10	_____	_____	_____
2. Attach electrode pads to the victim's bare dry chest as pictured on the AED. Place the electrodes at the sternum and apex of the heart. Make sure the pads are in complete contact with the victim's chest and that they do not overlap (see Figure 22-4).	20	_____	_____	_____
3. All rescuers must clear away from the victim. Press the Analyze button; the AED analyzes the victim's coronary status, announces whether the victim is going to be shocked, and automatically charges the electrodes.	20	_____	_____	_____
4. All rescuers must clear away from the victim. Press the SHOCK button if the machine is not automated. You may repeat 3 analyze-shock cyc.	20	_____	_____	_____
5. Deliver one shock; leave the AED attached and immediately perform CPR, starting with chest compressions.	10	_____	_____	_____
6. After five cycles of CPR (about 2 minutes), repeat the AED analysis and deliver another shock if indicated. If a nonshockable rhythm is detected, the AED should instruct the rescuer to resume CPR immediately, beginning with chest compressions.	10	_____	_____	_____
7. If the machine gives the "no shock indicated" signal, assess the victim. Check the carotid pulse and the person's breathing status and keep the AED attached until EMS arrives.	10	_____	_____	_____

351

Comments:

Points earned _____ ÷ 100 possible points = Score _____ % Score

Instructor's signature _____

PROCEDURE 22-7. PERFORM PATIENT SCREENING USING ESTABLISHED PROTOCOLS: TELEPHONE SCREENING AND APPROPRIATE DOCUMENTATION

CAAHEP COMPETENCIES: I.P.3., V.P.6., V.P.7.
ABHES COMPETENCIES: 8.f., 9.g.

TASK: Role-play the following scenario to assess the direction of emergency care and document information appropriately in the patient's record.

SCENARIO: Cheryl is working with the telephone screening staff when they receive a call from the mother of a 5-year-old patient. The mother reports that her son fell and cut his arm. What type of information should Cheryl gather about the injury? What action should be taken? How should the incident be documented?

EQUIPMENT AND SUPPLIES:
- Patient record
- Notepad and pen or pencil
- Facility's emergency procedures manual
- Computer scheduling program
- Area emergency numbers

Standards: Complete the procedure and all critical steps in _____ minutes with a minimum score of 85% in three attempts.

Scoring: Divide the points earned by the total possible points. Failure to perform a critical step, indicated by an asterisk (*), results in an unsatisfactory overall score.

Time began _____ **Time ended** _____ **Total minutes:** _____

Steps	Possible Points	Attempt 1	Attempt 2	Attempt 3
1. Stay calm and reassure the caller.	5	_____	_____	_____
2. Verify the identity of the caller and the injured patient.	5	_____	_____	_____
3. Immediately record the names of the caller and the patient, their location, and the phone number.	5	_____	_____	_____
*4. Determine whether the patient's condition is life threatening. Quantify the amount of blood loss and determine whether the patient is alert and responsive and breathing is normal. Notify EMS if necessary.	10	_____	_____	_____
5. If EMS is notified, stay on the line with the caller until EMS personnel arrive at the scene.	10	_____	_____	_____
*6. If emergency services are not needed, gather details about the injury to determine whether the patient can be seen in the office or should be referred to an emergency department (ED). Consider the following questions:	3	_____	_____	_____
a. Is there a suspected head or neck injury? Has the patient been moved?	3	_____	_____	_____
b. Is there a possible fracture? If so, where?	3	_____	_____	_____
c. Is bleeding present? Can it be easily controlled?	3	_____	_____	_____

Steps	Possible Points	Attempt 1	Attempt 2	Attempt 3
d. Are there any other symptoms?	3	_____	_____	_____
e. Is there anything pertinent in the patient's health history that would complicate the situation?	3	_____	_____	_____
f. Has the caller administered any first aid? If so, what type?	3	_____	_____	_____
7. Based on the information gathered, determine when the patient should be seen in the office if the person is not referred to an ED.	10	_____	_____	_____
*8. At any point in this process, do not hesitate to consult the provider or experienced staff or refer to the facility's emergency procedures manual to determine how to manage the patient's problem.	10	_____	_____	_____
9. Always allow the caller to hang up first, just in case more information or assistance is needed.	10	_____	_____	_____
*10. In the following Documentation in the Medical Record section, document as you would in the patient's record the information gathered, the actions taken or recommended, any home care recommendations, and whether the provider was notified.	14	_____	_____	_____

Documentation in the Medical Record

Comments:

Points earned _____ ÷ 100 possible points = **Score** _____ **% Score**

Instructor's signature _____

Name _____ Date _____ Score _____

PROCEDURE 22-8. MAINTAIN PROVIDER/PROFESSIONAL-LEVEL CPR CERTIFICATION: PERFORM ADULT RESCUE BREATHING AND ONE-RESCUER CPR; PERFORM PEDIATRIC AND INFANT CPR

CAAHEP COMPETENCIES: I.P.12.
ABHES COMPETENCIES: 9.g.

TASK: Restore a victim's breathing and circulation when respiration, pulse, or both stop.

EQUIPMENT AND SUPPLIES:
- Disposable gloves
- CPR ventilator mask for the adult, child, and infant
- Approved mannequins

Standards: Complete the procedure and all critical steps in _____ minutes with a minimum score of 85% in three attempts.

Scoring: Divide the points earned by the total possible points. Failure to perform a critical step, indicated by an asterisk (*), results in an unsatisfactory overall score.

Time began _____ Time ended _____ Total minutes: _____

Steps	Possible Points	Attempt 1	Attempt 2	Attempt 3
1. Establish unresponsiveness. Tap the victim and ask, "Are you OK?"	3	_____	_____	_____
2. If unresponsive, shout for help. Activate the emergency response system. Put on gloves and get a ventilator mask.	5	_____	_____	_____
3. Put the person on his or her back on a firm surface.	2	_____	_____	_____
4. If an AED is immediately available, deliver 1 shock if instructed by the device, then begin CPR.	2	_____	_____	_____
5. If an AED is immediately available, deliver 1 shock if instructed by the device, then begin CPR. If an AED is not available, check for breathing or only gasping to breathe while at the same time checking the carotid pulse for 10 seconds.	5	_____	_____	_____
*6. If there is no pulse, start chest compressions. Kneel at the victim's neck and shoulders a couple of inches away from the chest. Place the heel of the hand over the lower part of the sternum, between the nipples but above the xiphoid process.	3	_____	_____	_____
7. Place your other hand on top of the first and interlace or lift your fingers upward off the chest.	2	_____	_____	_____
*8. Bring your shoulders directly over the victim's sternum as you compress downward, keeping your elbows locked.	2	_____	_____	_____
*9. Use your upper body weight (not just your arms) as you push straight down on the sternum at least 2 inches but no more than 2.4 inches in an adult victim. Relax the pressure on the sternum after each compression, but do not remove your hands from the sternum.	5	_____	_____	_____

355

Steps	Possible Points	Attempt 1	Attempt 2	Attempt 3
*10. After performing 30 compressions (at a rate of about 100-120 compressions per minute), perform the head tilt–chin lift maneuver to open the airway. Tilt the victim's head by placing one hand on the forehead and applying enough pressure to push the head back; with the fingers of the other hand under the chin, lift up and pull the jaw forward. Look, listen, and feel for signs of breathing. Place your ear over the mouth and listen for breathing. Watch the rising and falling of the chest for evidence of breathing. If breathing is absent or inadequate, open the airway and place the ventilator mask over the victim's mouth and nose. Give 2 breaths (1 breath every 6 seconds—about 10 breaths per minute), holding the ventilator mask tightly against the face while tilting the victim's chin up to keep the airway open. Remove your mouth from the mouthpiece between breaths to allow time for the patient to exhale between breaths.	5	_____	_____	_____
*11. Check the patient's pulse (at the carotid artery for an adult or older child; at the brachial artery for an infant). If a pulse is present, continue rescue breathing (1 breath every 6 seconds—about 10 breaths per minute). If no signs of circulation are present, begin cycles of 30 chest compressions (at a rate of about 100-120 compressions per minute) followed by 2 breaths.	5	_____	_____	_____
12. If the person is still not responding after 5 cycles (about 2 minutes) and an AED is now available, apply it and follow the prompts. Administer 1 shock, then resume CPR, starting with chest compressions, for 2 more minutes before administering a second shock. Continue 30:2 cycles of compressions and ventilations. If an AED is not available, continue CPR until the person shows signs of movement or EMS personnel take over.	5	_____	_____	_____

Performing CPR on a child: The procedure for performing CPR on a child 1 to 8 years of age is essentially the same as that for an adult. The differences are as follows:

	Possible Points	Attempt 1	Attempt 2	Attempt 3
a. Perform 5 cycles of compressions and breaths on the child (30:2 ratio, about 2 minutes) before calling 911 or the local emergency number or using an AED. If another person is available, have that person activate EMS while you care for the child.	5	_____	_____	_____
b. Use only one hand to perform chest compressions.	2	_____	_____	_____
c. Breathe more gently.	2	_____	_____	_____
d. Use the same compression-to-breath ratio as used for adults, 30 compressions followed by 2 breaths per cycle; after 2 breaths, immediately begin the next cycle of compressions and breaths.	5	_____	_____	_____
e. After 5 cycles (about 2 minutes) of CPR without response, apply an AED if available. Use pediatric pads for children 1 to 8 years of age; if pediatric pads are not available, use adult pads. Do not use an AED on children younger than age 1. Administer 1 shock if instructed to do so, then resume CPR, starting with chest compressions, for 2 more minutes before administering a second shock.	5	_____	_____	_____
f. Continue until the child responds or help arrives.	3	_____	_____	_____

356

Steps	Possible Points	Attempt 1	Attempt 2	Attempt 3
Performing CPR on an infant: Infant cardiac arrest typically is caused by a lack of oxygen from drowning or choking. If you know the infant has an airway obstruction, clear the obstruction; if you do not know why the infant is unresponsive, perform CPR for 2 minutes (about 5 cycles) before calling 911 or the local emergency number. If another person is available, have that person call for help immediately while you attend to the baby.	5	_____	_____	_____
a. Draw an imaginary line between the infant's nipples. Place two fingers on the sternum just below this intermammary line.	3	_____	_____	_____
b. Gently compress the chest at a rate of 100-120 per minute.	4	_____	_____	_____
c. Administer 2 breaths after every 30 compressions.	3	_____	_____	_____
d. After about five 30:2 cycles, activate EMS.	3	_____	_____	_____
e. Continue CPR until the infant responds or help arrives.	3	_____	_____	_____
Rescue breathing for an infant:				
Use an infant ventilator mask or cover the baby's mouth and nose with your mouth.				
13. Give 2 rescue breaths by gently puffing out the cheeks and slowly breathing into the infant's mouth, taking about 1 second for each breath.	5	_____	_____	_____
14. Remove your gloves and the ventilator mask valve and discard them in the biohazard container. If the ventilator mask is not disposable, disinfect it per the manufacturer's recommendations. Sanitize your hands.	5	_____	_____	_____
*15. In the following Documentation in the Health Record section, document the procedure and the patient's condition as you would in the patient's health record.	5	_____	_____	_____

Comments:

Points earned _____ ÷ 100 possible points = Score _____ % Score

Instructor's signature _____

PROCEDURE 22-9. PERFORM FIRST AID PROCEDURES: ADMINISTER OXYGEN

CAAHEP COMPETENCIES: I.P.13.
ABHES COMPETENCIES: 9.g.

TASK: Provide oxygen for a patient in respiratory distress.

EQUIPMENT AND SUPPLIES:
- Provider's order
- Portable oxygen tank
- Pressure regulator
- Flow meter
- Nasal cannula with connecting tubing
- Patient's health record

Standards: Complete the procedure and all critical steps in _____ minutes with a minimum score of 85% in three attempts.

Scoring: Divide the points earned by the total possible points. Failure to perform a critical step, indicated by an asterisk (*), results in an unsatisfactory overall score.

Time began _____ Time ended _____ Total minutes: _____

Steps	Possible Points	Attempt 1	Attempt 2	Attempt 3
1. Gather equipment and sanitize your hands.	10	___	___	___
2. Greet and identify the patient, introduce yourself, and explain the procedure.	10	___	___	___
3. Check the pressure gauge on the tank to determine the amount of oxygen in the tank.	10	___	___	___
4. If necessary, open the cylinder on the tank one full counterclockwise turn; then attach the cannula tubing to the flow meter.	10	___	___	___
*5. Adjust the flow of oxygen according to the provider's order. Usually, the flow meter is set at 1-4 liters per minute (LPM). Check to make sure oxygen is flowing through the cannula.	20	___	___	___
*6. Insert the cannula tips into the patient's nostrils and adjust the tubing around the back of the ears.	10	___	___	___
*7. Encourage patient to breathe through nose with mouth closed.	5	___	___	___
*8. Make sure the patient is comfortable and answer any questions the patient may have.	10	___	___	___
9. Sanitize your hands.	5	___	___	___
*10. In the following Documentation in the Health Record section, document the procedure as you would in the patient's record. Include the number of liters of oxygen being administered and the patient's condition.	10	___	___	___

Comments:

Points earned _____ ÷ 100 possible points = **Score** _____ **% Score**

Instructor's signature _____

Name _____ Date _____ Score _____

PROCEDURE 22-10. PERFORM FIRST AID PROCEDURES: RESPOND TO AN AIRWAY OBSTRUCTION IN AN ADULT

CAAHEP COMPETENCIES: I.P.12., I.P.13.
ABHES COMPETENCIES: 9.g.

TASK: Remove an airway obstruction and restore ventilation.

EQUIPMENT AND SUPPLIES:
- Disposable gloves
- Ventilation mask (for unconscious victim)
- Approved mannequin for practicing removal of a foreign body airway obstruction (FBAO) in an unconscious person

Standards: Complete the procedure and all critical steps in _____ minutes with a minimum score of 85% in three attempts.

Scoring: Divide the points earned by the total possible points. Failure to perform a critical step, indicated by an asterisk (*), results in an unsatisfactory overall score.

Time began _____ Time ended _____ Total minutes: _____

Steps	Possible Points	Attempt 1	Attempt 2	Attempt 3
1. Ask the victim, "Are you choking?" If the victim indicates yes, ask, "Can you speak?" If the victim is unable to speak, tell the person you are going to help.	10	_____	_____	_____
2. Stand behind the victim with your feet slightly apart.	5	_____	_____	_____
3. Reach around the victim's abdomen and place an index finger into the victim's navel or at the level of the belt buckle. Make a fist of the opposite hand (do not tuck the thumb into the fist) and place the thumb side of the fist against the victim's abdomen above the navel. If the victim is pregnant, place the fist above the enlarged uterus. If the victim is obese, you may need to place the fist higher in the abdomen. (Chest thrusts may need to be performed on a pregnant or obese victim.)	10	_____	_____	_____
4. Place the opposite hand over the fist and give abdominal thrusts in a quick inward and upward movement.	10	_____	_____	_____
5. Repeat the abdominal thrusts until the object is expelled or the victim becomes unresponsive.	5	_____	_____	_____
Unresponsive Victim				
1. Carefully lower the patient to the ground, activate the emergency response system, and put on disposable gloves.	10	_____	_____	_____
2. Immediately begin CPR with 30 compressions and 2 breath cycles using the ventilator mask.	10	_____	_____	_____
3. Each time the airway is opened to deliver a rescue breath during CPR, look for an object in the victim's mouth and remove it if visible. If no object is found, immediately return to the cycle of 30 chest compressions.	10	_____	_____	_____

Chapter **22** **Safety and Emergency Practices**

Steps	Possible Points	Attempt 1	Attempt 2	Attempt 3
4. A finger sweep should be used only if the obstruction is visible.	5	_____	_____	_____
5. Continue cycles of 30 compressions to 2 rescue breaths until either the obstruction is removed or EMS arrives.	5	_____	_____	_____
6. If the obstruction is removed, assess the victim for breathing and circulation. If a pulse is present but the patient is not breathing, begin rescue breathing.	10	_____	_____	_____
7. Once the patient has been stabilized or EMS has taken over care, remove your gloves and the ventilator mask valve and discard them in the biohazard container. Disinfect the ventilator mask according to the manufacturer's recommendations. Sanitize your hands.	5	_____	_____	_____
8. In the following Documentation in the Health Record section, document the procedure and the patient's condition as you would in the patient's record.	5	_____	_____	_____

Documentation in the Health Record

Comments:

Points earned _____ ÷ 100 possible points = Score _____ % Score

Instructor's signature _____

Name _____ Date _____ Score _____

PROCEDURE 22-11. PERFORM FIRST AID PROCEDURES: CARE FOR A PATIENT WHO HAS FAINTED OR IS IN SHOCK

CAAHEP COMPETENCIES: I.P.13.e-f.
ABHES COMPETENCIES: 9.g.

TASK: Assess and provide emergency care for a patient who is in shock and has fainted.

EQUIPMENT AND SUPPLIES:
- Sphygmomanometer
- Stethoscope
- Watch with second hand
- Blanket
- Footstool or box
- Pillows
- Oxygen equipment, if ordered by the provider:
  - Portable oxygen tank
  - Pressure regulator
  - Flow meter
  - Nasal cannula with connecting tubing
- Patient's record

Standards: Complete the procedure and all critical steps in _____ minutes with a minimum score of 85% in three attempts.

Scoring: Divide the points earned by the total possible points. Failure to perform a critical step, indicated by an asterisk (*), results in an unsatisfactory overall score.

Time began _____ Time ended _____ Total minutes: _____

Steps	Possible Points	Attempt 1	Attempt 2	Attempt 3
*1. If a warning is given that the patient feels faint, have the patient lower the head to the knees to increase the blood supply to the brain. If this does not stop the episode, either have the patient lie down on the examination table or lower the patient to the floor. If the patient collapses to the floor when fainting, treat with caution because of possible head or neck injuries.	10	_____	_____	_____
*2. Immediately notify the provider of the patient's condition and assess the patient for life-threatening emergencies, such as respiratory or cardiac arrest. If the patient is breathing and has a pulse, monitor the vital signs.	10	_____	_____	_____
*3. If the patient has fainted and vital signs are unstable or the patient does not respond quickly, activate emergency medical services (EMS).	10	_____	_____	_____
*4. Activate EMS if the patient shows signs of shock—pale, gray, or cyanotic appearance; moist but cool skin; dilated pupils; a weak, rapid pulse; marked hypotension; shallow, rapid respirations; or lethargy or restlessness.	10	_____	_____	_____
*5. Look, listen, and feel for breathing and check the pulse. Maintain an open airway and continue to monitor vital signs.	10	_____	_____	_____

Steps	Possible Points	Attempt 1	Attempt 2	Attempt 3
*6. Loosen any tight clothing and keep the patient warm, applying a blanket if needed.	5	_____	_____	_____
*7. If a head or neck injury is not a factor, elevate the patient's legs above the level of the heart using a footstool with pillow support if available.	5	_____	_____	_____
8. Continue to monitor vital signs, and apply oxygen by nasal cannula if ordered by the provider until the patient recovers or EMS arrives.	10	_____	_____	_____
*9. If the patient vomits, roll the patient onto his or her side to prevent aspiration of vomitus into the lungs.	10	_____	_____	_____
10. If the patient completely recovers, assist the patient into a sitting position. Do not leave the patient unattended on the examination table.	10	_____	_____	_____
11. In the following Documentation in the Health Record section, document the incident as you would in the patient's record; include a description of the episode, the patient's symptoms and vital signs, the duration of the episode, and any complaints. If oxygen was administered, document the number of liters and how long oxygen was administered.	10	_____	_____	_____

Documentation in the Health Record

Comments:

Points earned _____ ÷ 100 possible points = Score _____ % Score

Instructor's signature _____

Name _____ Date _____ Score _____

PROCEDURE 22-12. PERFORM FIRST AID PROCEDURES: CARE FOR A PATIENT WITH SEIZURE ACTIVITY

CAAHEP COMPETENCIES: I.P.13.d.
ABHES COMPETENCIES: 9.g.

TASK: Assess and provide emergency care for a patient who has a grand mal seizure.

EQUIPMENT AND SUPPLIES:
- Patient's record
- Sphygmomanometer
- Stethoscope
- Watch with second hand
- Blanket
- Pillows

Standards: Complete the procedure and all critical steps in _____ minutes with a minimum score of 85% in three attempts.

Scoring: Divide the points earned by the total possible points. Failure to perform a critical step, indicated by an asterisk (*), results in an unsatisfactory overall score.

Time began _____ Time ended _____ Total minutes: _____

Steps	Possible Points	Attempt 1	Attempt 2	Attempt 3
*1. If warning is given that the patient might have a seizure, help lower the patient to the floor. If the patient collapses with a seizure, clear everything away from the patient that could cause accidental injury. If you cannot remove all hard items away (such as the examination table) pad the hard edges with a blanket or pillow.	10	_____	_____	_____
*2. Immediately check the time on your watch and call for help.	10	_____	_____	_____
*3. Observe the patient throughout the seizure but do not restrain or confine the patient's movements.	10	_____	_____	_____
*4. Do not place anything in the patient's mouth during the seizure.	10	_____	_____	_____
*5. After muscular contractions have ended, roll the patient into the recovery position on his side with the top knee bent and the head resting on the extended arm closest to the floor.	10	_____	_____	_____
*6. Loosen any tight clothing and keep the patient warm, using a blanket if needed. Let the patient rest, but never leave the patient alone.	10	_____	_____	_____
7. If the provider is not in the facility, check the policies and procedures manual to determine how to follow up with the patient.	10	_____	_____	_____

Steps	Possible Points	Attempt 1	Attempt 2	Attempt 3
8. Activate emergency medical services (EMS) if any of the following conditions are present:	10	_____	_____	_____

- The patient does not regain consciousness within 10 to 15 minutes.

- The seizure does not stop within a few minutes.

- The patient begins a second seizure immediately after the first one.

- The patient is pregnant.

- Signs of head trauma are present.

- The patient is known to have diabetes.

- The seizure was triggered by a high fever in a child.

Steps	Possible Points	Attempt 1	Attempt 2	Attempt 3
9. If the patient completely recovers, assist the patient into a sitting position, check vital signs, and make sure the patient has someone to accompany him or her home.	10	_____	_____	_____
*10. In the following Documentation in the Health Record section, document the incident, including a description of the episode, the patient's symptoms and vital signs, the duration of the seizure activity, and any complaints in the patient's record.	10	_____	_____	_____

Documentation in the Health Record

Comments:

Points earned _____ ÷ 100 possible points = **Score** _____ **% Score**

Instructor's signature _____

Name _____ Date _____ Score _____

PROCEDURE 22-13. PERFORM FIRST AID PROCEDURES: CARE FOR A PATIENT WITH A SUSPECTED FRACTURE OF THE WRIST BY APPLYING A SPLINT

CAAHEP COMPETENCIES: I.P.13.c.
ABHES COMPETENCIES: 9.g.

TASK: Provide emergency care for and assessment of a patient with a suspected fracture of the wrist.

EQUIPMENT AND SUPPLIES:
- Patient's record
- Sphygmomanometer
- Stethoscope
- Watch with second hand
- Splint with padding
- Ace or roller bandage material
- Gloves and sterile dressing if there are any open areas in the skin

Standards: Complete the procedure and all critical steps in _____ minutes with a minimum score of 85% in three attempts.

Scoring: Divide the points earned by the total possible points. Failure to perform a critical step, indicated by an asterisk (*), results in an unsatisfactory overall score.

Time began _____ Time ended _____ Total minutes: _____

Steps	Possible Points	Attempt 1	Attempt 2	Attempt 3
1. Gather equipment and sanitize your hands.	5	_____	_____	_____
2. Greet and identify the patient by full name and date of birth, introduce yourself, and explain the procedure.	5	_____	_____	_____
3. Obtain vital signs.	10	_____	_____	_____
*4. Assess the area of the suspected fracture for swelling, bleeding, bruising, or protruding bones.	10	_____	_____	_____
5. If the skin is broken, apply gloves and cover the area with a sterile dressing.	10	_____	_____	_____
*6. Moving the limb as little as possible, place the padded splint under the lower arm and wrist.	10	_____	_____	_____
*7. The area must be immobilized by the splint above and below the suspected fracture.	10	_____	_____	_____
*8. Secure the splint in place by rolling an Ace bandage or roller bandage around the splint and arm starting at the arm and rolling down to the wrist and hand.	10	_____	_____	_____
*9. Check the pulse in the affected arm; note the color and temperature of the skin and the color of the nails.	10	_____	_____	_____
10. Make sure the patient is comfortable, and answer any questions he or she may have.	5	_____	_____	_____

Steps	Possible Points	Attempt 1	Attempt 2	Attempt 3
11. Sanitize your hands.	5	_____	_____	_____
*12. In the following Documentation in the Health Record section, document the procedure including the condition of the patient, reported pain level, and application of the splint.	10	_____	_____	_____

Documentation in the Health Record

Comments:

Points earned _____ ÷ 100 possible points = Score _____ % Score

Instructor's signature _____

PROCEDURE 22-14. PERFORM FIRST AID PROCEDURES: CONTROL BLEEDING

CAAHEP COMPETENCIES: I.P.13.a.
ABHES COMPETENCIES: 9.g.

TASK: Stop hemorrhaging from an open wound.

EQUIPMENT AND SUPPLIES:
- Gloves (sterile if available)
- Appropriate personal protective equipment (PPE) according to OSHA guidelines, including:
  - Impermeable gown
  - Face shield or goggles
  - Impermeable mask
  - Impermeable foot covers if indicated
- Sterile dressings
- Bandaging material
- Biohazard waste container
- Patient's record

Standards: Complete the procedure and all critical steps in _____ minutes with a minimum score of 85% in three attempts.

Scoring: Divide the points earned by the total possible points. Failure to perform a critical step, indicated by an asterisk (*), results in an unsatisfactory overall score.

Time began _____ **Time ended** _____ **Total minutes:** _____

Steps	Possible Points	Attempt 1	Attempt 2	Attempt 3
*1. Sanitize your hands and put on the appropriate PPE.	10	_____	_____	_____
2. Assemble equipment and supplies.	10	_____	_____	_____
*3. Apply several layers of sterile dressing material directly to the wound and exert pressure.	10	_____	_____	_____
4. Wrap the wound with bandage material. Add more dressing and bandaging material if the bleeding continues.	10	_____	_____	_____
*5. If the bleeding persists and the wound is on an extremity, elevate the extremity above the level of the heart. Notify the provider immediately if the bleeding cannot be controlled.	10	_____	_____	_____
*6. If the bleeding still continues, maintain direct pressure and elevation; also apply pressure to the appropriate artery. If the wound is in the arm, apply pressure to the brachial artery by squeezing the inner aspect of the upper middle arm. If the wound is in the leg, apply pressure to the femoral artery on the affected side by pushing with the heel of the hand into the femoral crease at the groin. If the bleeding cannot be controlled, activate EMS.	15	_____	_____	_____
7. Once the bleeding has been brought under control and the patient has been stabilized, discard contaminated materials in an appropriate biohazard waste container.	10	_____	_____	_____

Steps	Possible Points	Attempt 1	Attempt 2	Attempt 3
8. Disinfect the area, remove your gloves, and discard them in the biohazard waste container.	10	_____	_____	_____
9. Sanitize your hands.	5	_____	_____	_____
*10. In the following Documentation in the Health Record section, document the incident as you would in the patient's record; include the details of the wound, when and how it occurred, the patient's symptoms and vital signs, the treatment provided by the provider, and the patient's current condition.	10	_____	_____	_____

Documentation in the Health Record

Comments:

Points earned _____ **÷ 100 possible points = Score** _____ **% Score**

Instructor's signature _____

Name _____ Date _____ Score _____

PROCEDURE 22-15. PERFORM FIRST AID PROCEDURES: CARE FOR A PATIENT WITH A DIABETIC EMERGENCY

CAAHEP COMPETENCIES: I.P.13.b.
ABHES COMPETENCIES: 9.g.

TASK: Provide emergency care for and assessment of a patient with insulin shock or a pending diabetic coma. Students should take turns role-playing a diabetic patient with hypoglycemia, hyperglycemia, and the medical assistant.

EQUIPMENT AND SUPPLIES:
- Patient's record
- Sphygmomanometer
- Stethoscope
- Watch with second hand
- Disposable gloves
- Glucometer
- Disposable lancet
- Glucose tablets
- Insulin
- Insulin syringe unit
- Alcohol swabs
- Sharps container

Standards: Complete the procedure and all critical steps in _____ minutes with a minimum score of 85% in three attempts.

Scoring: Divide the points earned by the total possible points. Failure to perform a critical step, indicated by an asterisk (*), results in an unsatisfactory overall score.

Time began _____ Time ended _____ Total minutes: _____

Steps	Possible Points	Attempt 1	Attempt 2	Attempt 3
1. Gather equipment and sanitize your hands.	5	____	____	____
2. Greet and identify the patient; introduce yourself.	5	____	____	____
3. Obtain vital signs.	10	____	____	____
*4. If the patient is known to have diabetes, observe for signs and symptoms that indicate a diabetic emergency.	10			
a. Signs and symptoms of insulin shock or hypoglycemia: rapid onset of vertigo, fatigue, hunger, tachycardia, profuse sweating, headache, irritability, seizures, and coma.		____	____	____
b. Signs and symptoms of impending diabetic coma or hyperglycemia: Symptoms develop more slowly than those of insulin shock; these include general malaise, dry mouth, polyuria, polydipsia, nausea, vomiting, shortness of breath (SOB), and breath with an acetone (or "fruity") smell.		____	____	____
*5. Immediately report patient's condition to the provider and follow his or her orders.	5	____	____	____

Steps	Possible Points	Attempt 1	Attempt 2	Attempt 3
*6. In an emergency situation, if a patient diagnosed with diabetes mellitus shows signs and symptoms of a diabetic emergency, the patient should be given glucose.	5	_____	_____	_____
*7. Follow the provider's orders and administer 15 g of carbohydrate immediately, preferably in the form of glucose tablets because they have a known concentrated quantity of glucose. If glucose tablets are not available, give the patient ½ cup of fruit juice or 5 or 6 pieces of hard candy.	10	_____	_____	_____
*8. Check the patient's blood glucose levels with a glucometer and monitor vital signs.	10	_____	_____	_____
• If the blood glucose level is below 80 mg/dL (insulin shock), administer another 15 g of carbohydrate. Wait 15 minutes and check the glucometer reading again. If the level is still low, repeat steps 7 and 8.				
• If the patient's blood glucose levels are elevated (diabetic coma) administer insulin as ordered by the provider.				
*9. Continue to monitor the patient and follow the provider's orders regarding continued care.	10	_____	_____	_____
• A patient with insulin shock can be stabilized by continued monitoring of blood glucose and administration of glucose every 15 minutes until levels reach normal.				
• A patient with pending diabetic coma may need to be transported to the hospital.				
10. Dispose of used supplies and gloves in the appropriate biohazard containers (sharps containers for used lancets and injection unit).	5	_____	_____	_____
11. Sanitize your hands.	5	_____	_____	_____
*12. In the following Documentation in the Health Record section, document the actions taken and the patient's condition including vital signs, glucometer readings, administration of glucose or insulin, and whether the patient was stabilized and discharged or EMS was activated and the patient was transported to the hospital.	10	_____	_____	_____

Documentation in the Health Record

Comments:

Points earned _____ ÷ 100 possible points = Score _____ **% Score**

Instructor's signature _____

23 Career Development and Life Skills

VOCABULARY REVIEW

Fill in the blanks with the correct vocabulary terms from this chapter.

1. Before advertising a job posting, the employer needs to identify the _____ _____ or abilities required for the position.

2. June wanted to pay back her student loan and not _____ on it.

3. Debby needed to _____ her résumé and cover letter before she e-mailed them to the potential employer.

4. Sally and her classmates were able to practice their interviewing skills as they participated in a(n) _____ interview.

5. Jim joined the local medical assistant chapter so he could start _____ before graduation.

6. The employer required strong soft skills or _____ _____ for the medical assistant position.

7. Michaela made a(n) _____ for the receptionist position she was offered.

8. Christi watched the local _____ _____ for the type of position she wanted.

SKILLS AND CONCEPTS

Part I: Short Answer

1. List three reasons a graduating medical assistant should take advantage of job search training.

   a. _____
   b. _____
   c. _____

2. What are the personality traits that are most important to employers?

   a. _____
   b. _____
   c. _____
   d. _____

3. List four interpersonal skills that are crucial in today's fast-paced healthcare environment.

   a. _____
   b. _____
   c. _____
   d. _____

373

4. Describe five ways a person can demonstrate professionalism.

    a. _____

    b. _____

    c. _____

    d. _____

    e. _____

5. Define *technical skills* and give two examples.

_____

_____

6. Define *transferable job skills* and give two examples.

_____

_____

7. What is meant when it is said that a medical assistant knows his or her personal needs?

_____

_____

8. List and define the two best job search methods.

    a. _____

    b. _____

9. Explain two ways a person can be organized in his or her job search.

    a. _____

    b. _____

10. List three types of résumés and describe why each is used.

    a. _____

    b. _____

    c. _____

11. Describe the purpose of a career portfolio.

_____

_____

12. Describe three ways a medical assistant can prepare for an interview.

    a. _____

    b. _____

    c. _____

13. List and discuss three legal applicant interview questions.

    a. _____

    b. _____

    c. _____

14. List and discuss three illegal applicant interview questions.

a. _____

b. _____

c. _____

Part II: Résumé, Cover Letter, and Application

Job Postings:

Medical Assistant Position–Full Time (#23493)

Seeking a highly motivated, energetic, and dependable individual to join our health care facility. This individual must have the ability to work productively and effectively in a fast-paced environment. Responsibilities would include rooming patients (obtaining vital signs and medical history) and recording information in patients' electronic chart. Must have exceptional computer skills and excellent interpersonal skills (communication and customer service skills), with the ability to interact professionally with patients, physicians, and co-workers in a calm and efficient manner. Must be a graduate of an accredited medical assistant program and pass a national medical assistant exam within 6 months of hire.

Receptionist Position–Full Time (#23494)

Seeking a highly motivated, energetic, organized, and dependable individual to join our health care facility. This individual must have the ability to work productively and effectively in a fast-paced environment. Responsibilities would include answering phones, managing appointments using an electronic scheduling system, creating correspondence to patients and providers, and greeting patients. Must have exceptional computer skills and excellent interpersonal skills (communication and customer service skills), with the ability to interact professionally with patients, physicians, and co-workers in a calm and efficient manner. Must have a high school diploma or equivalent. College education preferred.

Send your application and résumé to the address or e-mail below:

Attention: (your instructor's name)   Email: (your instructor's e-mail address)

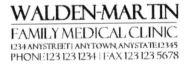

WALDEN-MARTIN
FAMILY MEDICAL CLINIC
1234 ANYSTREET | ANYTOWN, ANYSTATE 12345
PHONE 123 123 1234 | FAX 123 123 5678

1. Select one of the job postings or use a real job posting. Circle the key words that should be incorporated into the cover letter and/or résumé.

2. For the selected job posting, write a professional chronologic résumé. Incorporate some of the key phrases in your résumé. Use the suggestions in the textbook and follow Procedure 23-1 Prepare a Chronologic Résumé.

3. For the selected job posting, write a cover letter. Incorporate some of the key phrases in your letter. Use the suggestions in the textbook and follow Procedure 23-2 Create a Cover Letter.

4. For the selected job posting, complete the application. Incorporate some of the key phrases in the application. Use the suggestions in the textbook and follow Procedure 23-3 Complete a Job Application.

Part III: Career Portfolio

For these activities, refer to the selected job posting from Part II.

1. Plan how you would assemble your career portfolio. Complete the table, adding in the main topic areas and then identify the documents you would include.

Name of Main Areas (Tabbed Sections of Portfolio)	List Documents That Provide Positive Support of Your Skill Set and Knowledge

2. For the selected job posting, create a career portfolio. Incorporate documents that emphasize the key phrases identified in the posting. Use the suggestions in the textbook and follow Procedure 23-4 Create a Career Portfolio.

Part IV: Interviews

For these activities, refer to the selected job posting from Part II unless an actual interview is set up.

1. Describe what you would wear to an interview. Be specific and describe the articles of clothing you would wear.

_____

_____

2. Describe what activities you would do before the interview to prepare yourself for the interview.

_____

_____

3. Answer the following common interview questions. Use complete sentences and proper grammar. Your answers should include at least 5 sentences.

   a. "Tell us about yourself."

   b. "Why do you want to work at this clinic?"

   c. "Why should we hire you?"

   d. "How do you work under pressure? Please give us an example of a past experience you have had."

   e. "How do you handle criticism? Please give us an example of a past experience you have had."

   f. "What do you think your co-workers think or would say about you?"

Chapter 23 Career Development and Life Skills

Copyright © 2017 Elsevier, Inc. All rights reserved.

g. "Describe your last supervisor."

h. "How would you describe the perfect job?"

i. "Why did you choose this type of profession?"

j. "Describe two of your strongest qualities."

k. "Describe two of your weakest qualities."

l. "Where do you see yourself in 5 years? 10 years?"

m. "What questions do you have for us?"

4. Attend a real or mock interview. (A mock interview can use peers or instructors as the interviewers.) Prepare yourself for the mock interview using the suggestions in the textbook. During the interview, follow Procedure 23-5 Practice Interview Skills during a Mock Interview.

Part V: Follow-Up Activities

For these activities, refer to the selected job posting from Part II unless an actual interview is set up.

1. Describe the appropriate ways of following up after an interview.

_____

_____

2. Describe the importance of sending a thank-you note after an interview.

_____

_____

3. For the selected job posting and interview, create a thank-you note. Use the suggestions in the textbook and follow Procedure 23-6 Create a Thank-you Note for an Interview.

Part VI: You Got the Job

1. What is the purpose of the probationary period?

_____

_____

2. Describe how you could be a good employee.

_____

_____

3. What is the purpose of the performance appraisal?

_____

_____

4. Describe how to leave a job.

_____

_____

Part VII: Life Skills

1. Describe the term *personal growth.*

_____

_____

2. Why is having good self-esteem important to a healthcare professional?

_____

_____

3. Why is having strong decision-making skills important for a healthcare professional?

_____

_____

4. Describe the importance of professional development for a healthcare professional?

_____

_____

5. Describe the importance of using positive stress management techniques.

_____

_____

6. List six positive stress management techniques.

a. _____

b. _____

c. _____

d. _____

e. _____

f. _____

CASE STUDY

Monica was an exceptional student during school and graduated with a high grade point average. After a successful practicum and 1 month looking for employment, she has been unable to secure a job. She calls the placement officer at her school, who sends her on several interviews, which are also unsuccessful. The placement officer asks Monica to come to the school dressed for an interview and to bring her résumé. The placement officer is impressed with Monica's appearance and her communication skills during the interview. However, when she looks down at Monica's résumé, she realizes why Monica has not been hired.

Monica Smith
1222 oak way, Mytown, OH 45458
Cell: 711-555-1253
Email: one_hot_chick@elsevier.net

Objective
I want to get a medical assistant daytime job, where I can get a high salary and not have to work weekends or holidays.

Education
Community College, Mytown, OH
Medical Assistant Diploma, 20XX

Health Care Experience
Family Practice Associates, Mytown, oh
Medical Assistant Practicum, April to May 20XX (220 hours)
I did a lot of jobs for my mentor like cleaning rooms and rooming patients.

Work Experience
Mytown Family Dinner, Mytown, OH
Cook
I cooked food for the customers and cleaned up the kitchen.

Special Skills
Keyboarding speed: 43 wpm

Credentials
Certified Medical Assistant, American Association of Medical Assistants (expires June 20XX)
BLS for Healthcare Providers, American Heart Association (expires September 20XX)

Hobbies
Riding horseback
Watching old movies

1. Describe at least four issues with the résumé that might cause Monica not to be hired. For each issue you describe, explain what Monica can do to be more likely to secure employment.

a. _____
_____

b. _____
_____

c. _____
_____

d. _____
_____

WORKPLACE ACTIVITY OPTION

1. Make a list of 20 potential employers. Include the title of potential positions that interest you and their job posting board website.

2. Submit the application and a résumé if you are close to the end of your training.

379

INTERNET ACTIVITIES

Complete one or more of these activities and share your results with the class, if appropriate.

1. Use the Internet to locate potential job opportunities. Have your résumé in electronic format ready to attach so that you can apply for the jobs that interest you.

2. Look for job search sites other than those in the textbook. Share the sites with your classmates.

3. Form a group on a social networking site, such as Facebook, that includes each classmate. Share e-mails and stay in touch with one another after graduation. Share leads that might result in employment.

4. Perform a job search for medical assistant positions in your area. Look for the 15 most interesting opportunities and print the job descriptions. Compare the job requirements to the skills you have learned. If appropriate, apply for the positions.

PROCEDURE 23-1. PREPARE A CHRONOLOGIC RÉSUMÉ

ABHES COMPETENCIES: 11.a.

TASK: Write an effective résumé for use as a tool in obtaining employment.

EQUIPMENT AND SUPPLIES:
- Computer with word processing software and a printer
- Current job posting
- Résumé paper
- Paper and pen

Standards: Complete the procedure and all critical steps in _____ minutes with a minimum score of 85% within three attempts.

Scoring: Divide the points earned by the total possible points. Failure to perform a critical step, indicated by an asterisk (*), results in an unsatisfactory overall score.

Time began _____ **Time ended** _____ **Total minutes:** _____

Steps	Possible Points	Attempt 1	Attempt 2	Attempt 3
1. Apply critical thinking skills as you create a list of the personality traits, technical skills, and transfer job skills that you possess. Also write down your career goal(s).	5	_____	_____	_____
2. Using the current job posting, identify the required and recommended qualifications and credentials needed for the position.	5	_____	_____	_____
3. Using the computer with word processing software, create a professional appearing header in the document's header. Include your name, address, telephone number(s), and e-mail address. Select an appropriate font style for your name and a smaller font size for your contact information.	10	_____	_____	_____
4. In the body of the document, create a section header for "Objective" and type a concise sentence stating your employment objective or goals. These goals should relate to the position being advertised.	10	_____	_____	_____
5. Create a section header for "Education." For the learning institution(s) you attended, list the school's name, city and state, degree obtained or coursework successfully completed, and the year. Include any additional educational information, like GPA, awards, and practicum information.	10	_____	_____	_____
6. Create a section header for your work experience. Provide details about your work experience, including the agency's name, city and state, title of your position, start and end date (month and year), and job duties. The job duties must start with an active verb using the appropriate tense.	10	_____	_____	_____
7. Create a section header for "Special Skills" and list your special language skills, computer proficiencies, and other notable skills you possess that relate to the position.	10	_____	_____	_____

Steps	Possible Points	Attempt 1	Attempt 2	Attempt 3
8. Create a section header for "Certifications and Credentials" and list the active credentials and certifications you have. Include the title of the certification, awarding agency, and the expiration date.	10	_____	_____	_____
9. All information on the résumé needs to appear in reverse chronologic order (newest information is on top).	10	_____	_____	_____
10. The résumé needs to look professional and interesting. Use font styles (bold, underline, italic font) to highlight important words and phrases. Use professional-looking bullets to list job duties and other information. Use the key words from the posting throughout the résumé.	10	_____	_____	_____
11. Proofread the résumé. Correct any spelling, grammar, punctuation, or sentence structure errors you find. If time allows, have another person review the résumé and use the feedback to revise your résumé.	5	_____	_____	_____
12. Print the résumé on résumé paper and proofread one final time. Any errors should be corrected and the document should be reprinted or e-mailed to the instructor.	5	_____	_____	_____

Comments:

Points earned _____ ÷ 100 possible points = **Score** _____ **% Score**

Instructor's signature _____

Name _____ Date _____ Score _____

MAERB/CAAHEP COMPETENCIES: V.P.8.
ABHES COMPETENCIES: 11.a.

TASK: Write an effective cover letter that will accompany the résumé.

EQUIPMENT AND SUPPLIES:
- Computer with word processing software and a printer
- Current job posting
- Résumé paper
- Paper and pen

Standards: Complete the procedure and all critical steps in _____ minutes with a minimum score of 85% within three attempts.

Scoring: Divide the points earned by the total possible points. Failure to perform a critical step, indicated by an asterisk (*), results in an unsatisfactory overall score.

Time began _____ Time ended _____ Total minutes: _____

Steps	Possible Points	Attempt 1	Attempt 2	Attempt 3
1. Using the job posting, read through the job description. With a pen, circle the position requirements and the key phrases.	5	_____	_____	_____
2. Using the computer with word processing software, create a professional-appearing header in the document's header that matches your résumé header. Include your name, address, telephone number(s), and e-mail address.	10	_____	_____	_____
3. Type the date in the correct location using the correct format. Have one blank line between the date line and the last line of the letterhead.	10	_____	_____	_____
4. Type the inside address using the correct spelling, punctuation, and location for the information. Leave 1-9 blank lines between the date and the inside address, depending on the location of the body of the letter.	10	_____	_____	_____
5. Starting on the second line below the inside address, type the salutation using the correct professional format, including the individual's name if known.	10	_____	_____	_____
6. Type the message in the body of the letter using the proper location and format. There should be a blank line after the salutation and between each paragraph. The message should be clear, concise, and professional. Use proper grammar, punctuation, capitalization, and sentence structure.	10	_____	_____	_____
7. The first paragraph should contain the title and number of the job posting. The middle paragraph(s) should summarize your strengths and include key phrases from the posting. The final paragraph should discuss your availability for an interview. The body should end with an expression of gratitude to the reader.	10	_____	_____	_____

Steps	Possible Points	Attempt 1	Attempt 2	Attempt 3
8. Type a proper closing, leaving one blank line between the last line of the body and the closing. Use the correct format and location.	10	_____	_____	_____
9. Type the signature block using the correct format and location. There should be four blank lines between the closing and the signature block.	10	_____	_____	_____
10. Spell check and proofread the document. Check for proper tone, grammar, punctuation, capitalization- and sentence structure. Check for proper spacing between the parts of the letter.	10	_____	_____	_____
11. Make any final corrections. Print the document on résumé paper and sign the letter or e-mail the document to your instructor.	5	_____	_____	_____

Comments:

Points earned _____ ÷ 100 possible points = Score _____ % Score

Instructor's signature _____

Name _____ Date _____ Score _____

PROCEDURE 23-3. COMPLETE A JOB APPLICATION

ABHES COMPETENCIES: 11.a.

TASK: Complete an accurate, detailed job application legibly to secure a job offer.

EQUIPMENT AND SUPPLIES:
- Pen
- Application form (Work Product 23-1 Application Form)
- Information regarding your past education, job experiences, and skill set you have obtained
- Contact information for former supervisors and references
- Current résumé

Standards: Complete the procedure and all critical steps in _____ minutes with a minimum score of 85% within three attempts.

Scoring: Divide the points earned by the total possible points. Failure to perform a critical step, indicated by an asterisk (*), results in an unsatisfactory overall score.

Time began _____ Time ended _____ Total minutes: _____

Steps	Possible Points	Attempt 1	Attempt 2	Attempt 3
1. Read the entire job application before completing any part of the document.	5	_____	_____	_____
2. Refer to your information on past jobs, education experiences, and skill sets you have obtained as you complete the application. Answers to the questions need to be accurate and honest.	60	_____	_____	_____
3. Use proper grammar, sentence structure, punctuation, spelling, and capitalization. Handwriting should be legible to the reader.	5	_____	_____	_____
4. Do not leave any space blank. Answer each question on the document. If the question does not apply, write "not applicable."	5	_____	_____	_____
5. Do not write "see résumé" anywhere on the document.	5	_____	_____	_____
6. Include information on the application that exhibits dependability, punctuality, teamwork, attention to detail, positive work ethics and initiative, the ability to adapt to change, a responsible attitude, and use of technology.	10	_____	_____	_____
7. Sign the document and date it.	5	_____	_____	_____
8. Proofread the document and make sure none of the information conflicts with the résumé.	5	_____	_____	_____

Comments:

Points earned _____ ÷ 100 possible points = Score _____ % Score

Instructor's signature _____

Name _____ Date _____ Score _____

PROCEDURE 23-4. CREATE A CAREER PORTFOLIO

ABHES COMPETENCIES: 11.a.

TASK: Create a custom portfolio that provides potential employers evidence of your skills and knowledge as a medical assistant.

EQUIPMENT AND SUPPLIES:
- Three-ring binder or folder
- Plastic sleeves for the 3-ring binder
- Dividers with tabs for the 3-ring binder
- Current résumé and cover letter
- Documents providing evidence of your skills and knowledge (transcripts, job and practicum evaluation forms, practicum skill checklist, projects completed in school, letters of recommendation, copies of certifications [CPR and First Aid cards])

Standards: Complete the procedure and all critical steps in _____ minutes with a minimum score of 85% within three attempts.

Scoring: Divide the points earned by the total possible points. Failure to perform a critical step, indicated by an asterisk (*), results in an unsatisfactory overall score.

Time began _____ Time ended _____ Total minutes: _____

Steps	Possible Points	Attempt 1	Attempt 2	Attempt 3
1. Group documents in a logical manner, putting like documents together. Identify the arrangement for the portfolio. You may want to include a table of contents to identify the tabbed areas.	40	_____	_____	_____
2. Neatly write the topic area on the tab of the dividers.	10	_____	_____	_____
3. Place the documents in plastic pockets, with one document per pocket.	10	_____	_____	_____
4. Arrange the documents neatly in the binder or folder. Have your cover letter and résumé in the front of all the other documents.	30	_____	_____	_____
5. After the portfolio is assembled, review the entire portfolio to ensure that it looks professional and the documents provide positive support of your skill set and knowledge.	10	_____	_____	_____

Comments:

Points earned _____ + 100 possible points = Score _____ % Score

Instructor's signature _____

PROCEDURE 23-5. PRACTICE INTERVIEW SKILLS DURING A MOCK INTERVIEW

ABHES COMPETENCIES: 11.a.

TASKS: Project a professional appearance during a job interview and express the reasons the medical assistant is the best candidate for the position.

EQUIPMENT AND SUPPLIES:
- Current job posting
- Résumé
- Cover letter
- Interview portfolio (optional)
- Application (optional)
- Interviewer
- Mock interview questions

Standards: Complete the procedure and all critical steps in _____ minutes with a minimum score of 85% within three attempts.

Scoring: Divide the points earned by the total possible points. Failure to perform a critical step, indicated by an asterisk (*), results in an unsatisfactory overall score.

Time began _____ Time ended _____ Total minutes: _____

Steps	Possible Points	Attempt 1	Attempt 2	Attempt 3
1. Presents wearing interview-appropriate attire and groomed professionally.	15	_____	_____	_____
2. Portrays a professional image by shaking hands firmly and bringing a copy of current résumé, cover letter, and copies of earned certificates. No visible nervous habits such as tapping feet, bouncing a crossed leg, drumming fingers, etc.	15	_____	_____	_____
3. Answers introductory question by providing only professional information.	10	_____	_____	_____
4. Answers interview questions with open, honest, and positive responses. Completely answers questions, provides information, and does not answer in single sentences or limited responses.	30	_____	_____	_____
5. Uses key words from job posting while answering interview questions.	10	_____	_____	_____
6. Asks interviewer 2-3 appropriate questions about the agency or the position.	10	_____	_____	_____
7. Expresses interest in the job and politely completes the interview by shaking hands and thanking the interviewer for the opportunity for the interview.	10	_____	_____	_____

Comments:

Points earned _____ ÷ 100 possible points = **Score** _____ **% Score**

Instructor's signature _____

Name _____ Date _____ Score _____

PROCEDURE 23-6. CREATE A THANK-YOU NOTE FOR AN INTERVIEW

ABHES COMPETENCIES: 11.a.

TASK: Create a meaningful thank-you note to be sent after the interview process.

EQUIPMENT AND SUPPLIES:
- Computer with word processing software
- Job description
- Contact name from interview

Standards: Complete the procedure and all critical steps in _____ minutes with a minimum score of 85% within three attempts.

Scoring: Divide the points earned by the total possible points. Failure to perform a critical step, indicated by an asterisk (*), results in an unsatisfactory overall score.

Time began _____ **Time ended** _____ **Total minutes:** _____

Steps	Possible Points	Attempt 1	Attempt 2	Attempt 3
1. Compose a professional letter using business letter format and word processing software. Include all of the required elements in the letter. Use correct spacing between the elements.	50	_____	_____	_____
2. Highlight the particulars of the interview in the body of the letter.	10	_____	_____	_____
3. Cover positive information you wish you had covered in the interview.	25	_____	_____	_____
4. Create a message that is concise and to the point.	10	_____	_____	_____
5. Sign and send the thank-you note.	5	_____	_____	_____

Comments:

Points earned _____ ÷ 100 possible points = Score _____ % Score

Instructor's signature _____

Name: _____

WORK PRODUCT 23-1. JOB APPLICATION

Corresponds to PROCEDURE 23-3

ABHES COMPETENCIES: 11.a.

WALDEN-MARTIN
FAMILY MEDICAL CLINIC
1234 ANYSTREET | ANYTOWN, ANYSTATE 12345
PHONE 123 123 1234 | FAX 123 123 5678

APPLICATION FOR EMPLOYMENT

Walden-Martin Family Medical Clinic is an equal opportunity employer and upholds the principles of equal opportunity employment. It is the policy of Walden-Martin Family Medical Clinic to provide employment, compensation and other benefits related to employment based on qualifications and performance, without regard to race, color, religion, national origin, age, sex, veteran status or disability, or any other basis prohibited by federal or state law. As an equal opportunity employer, Walden-Martin Family Medical Clinic intends to comply fully with all federal and state laws, and the information requested on this application will not be used for any purpose prohibited by law. Disabled applicants may request any needed accommodation. Please complete this application using ink, answer all questions completely, and sign the application.

Date: _____

Name: (First, Middle Initial, Last) _____

Social Security No.: _____   Phone: _____

Address: _____

City, State, Zip: _____

Have you been previously employed by Walden-Martin Family Medical Clinic?
☐ Yes ☐ No

If "Yes", when and job title?

How did you learn of the position for which you are applying?

☐ Newspaper/Print Advertisement ☐ Friend/Relative ☐ Employment Agency
☐ Job Service
☐ Radio/TV Advertisement ☐ Clinic Staff Person Name:

EMPLOYMENT DESIRED

Position(s) applied for: _____

☐ Full-time ☐ Part-time (If "Part time", number of shifts/hours desired _____)

Date available to start: _____ Salary requested: _____

PERSONAL HISTORY

Are you a United States citizen or do you have an entry permit which allows you to lawfully work in the U.S.? ☐ Yes ☐ No
 If applicable, Visa Type: _____ Immigration No.: _____

Are you at least 18 years old? ☐ Yes ☐ No

Are you ineligible to be employed with an AnyState licensed health care entity as a result of being found guilty by a court of law for abusing, neglecting, or mistreating individuals in a health care related setting? ☐ Yes ☐ No
 If "Yes," please explain: _____

Are you able to perform all of the duties required by the position for which you are applying, without endangering yourself or compromising the safety, health, or welfare of the patients or other staff member? ☐ Yes ☐ No
 If "No," please explain:_____

EDUCATION

	Name, City, State	Graduation Date	Course of Study/ Degree Obtained
High School:			
College:			
Other:			

LICENSURE/CERTIFICATION/REGISTRATION

Type of Certification, License or Registration	Agency/State	Registration Name

List any special skills or qualifications which you possess and feel are relevant to health care and the position for which you are applying.

_____

_____

_____

_____

_____

MILITARY SERVICE

From: _____ To: _____

Branch: _____

Duties: _____

Did you receive any specialized training? ☐ Yes ☐ No
If "Yes", describe: _____

EMPLOYMENT HISTORY

Please give accurate and complete information. Start with present or most recent employer.
May we contact and communicate with your present employer? ☐ Yes   ☐ No

Employer:		Phone:	
Address:		Supervisor:	
Employed	Start: Month/Year: _____ Ended: Month/Year: _____	Hourly Pay:	Start: _____ Ended: _____
Position title and responsibilities:			
Reason for leaving:			

Employer:		Phone:	
Address:		Supervisor:	
Employed	Start: Month/Year: _____ Ended: Month/Year: _____	Hourly Pay:	Start: _____ Ended: _____
Position title and responsibilities:			
Reason for leaving:			

Employer:		Phone:	
Address:		Supervisor:	
Employed	Start: Month/Year: _____ Ended: Month/Year: _____	Hourly Pay:	Start: _____ Ended: _____
Position title and responsibilities:			
Reason for leaving:			

Employer:		Phone:	
Address:		Supervisor:	
Employed	Start: Month/Year: _____ Ended: Month/Year: _____	Hourly Pay:	Start: _____ Ended: _____
Position title and responsibilities:			
Reason for leaving:			

REFERENCES

Names of co-workers (no relatives) you have worked with and whom we may contact for a reference.

Name:	
Address:	
Phone:	
Job Title:	

Name:	
Address:	
Phone:	
Job Title:	

Name:	
Address:	
Phone:	
Job Title:	

Please read the following statements completely and carefully before you sign your name.

The Applicant HEREBY CERTIFIES that the answers given on this Application For Employment, including any statements or answers provided by the Applicant during interview, are true and correct. The Applicant fully authorizes Walden-Martin Family Medical Clinic to contact any references, past and present employers, persons, schools, law enforcement agencies and any other sources of information which may be relevant to the Applicant and this Application For Employment. It is understood and agreed that any misrepresentation, false statement, or omission by the Applicant will be sufficient reason for rejection of the Application For Employment or for dismissal from employment at any time, without recourse or liability to Walden-Martin Family Medical Clinic.

I have read, understand and agree to the above statement.

Sign: _____

Date: _____